# The Galveston Diet Cookbook for beginners

Nourishing Your Body, Balancing Hormones, and Embracing a Healthy Lifestyle with Wholesome and Delicious Recipes

By

Grace M. Bennett

# Table of contents

Sweet Potato and Kale Soup

Tomato Basil Quinoa Soup

Coconut Curry Chickpea Stew

Lemon Garlic Chickpea Stew

Cabbage and White Bean Soup

Miso Vegetable Soup

Cajun Black-Eyed Pea Soup

Thai Coconut Pumpkin Soup

**Conclusion**

# Introduction

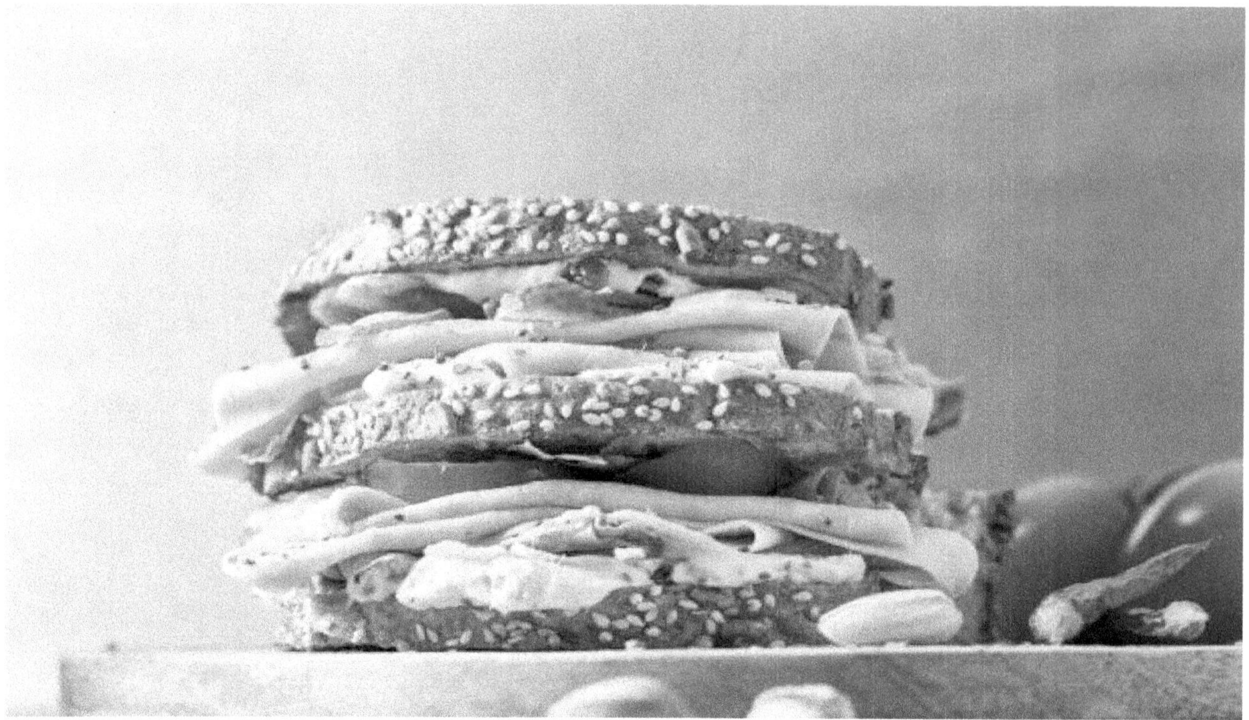

Welcome to "The Galveston Diet Cookbook for Beginners," your starting point on a transformative journey to fuel your body, balance your hormones, and adopt a healthy lifestyle. This cookbook is more than simply a collection of recipes; it's a guide to rethinking your relationship with food and promoting overall health.

This cookbook, created in accordance with The Galveston Diet principles, is intended for those who want not only delicious and enjoyable meals, but also a holistic approach to health. Whether you're a seasoned cook or just starting out, these recipes are designed to make your experience pleasurable and rewarding.

The next sections provide a wide variety of recipes for breakfasts, snacks, appetizers, vegetables, sides, fish, shellfish, beef, pork, lamb, chicken, desserts, soups, and stews. Each recipe is carefully crafted to provide a balanced blend of flavors while keeping to the principles that constitute The Galveston Diet.

As you engage on this culinary adventure, keep in mind that The Galveston Diet is a lifestyle centered on full, nutrient-dense foods rather than a rigid routine. It's about finding balance, listening to your body, and enjoying the road to peak health.

This cookbook is your guide to achieving hormonal balance, weight management, or simply a more vibrant and energetic life. Prepare to embark on a savory trip that extends beyond the plate, nurturing your body, mind, and spirit.

Allow the pages of "The Galveston Diet Cookbook for Beginners" to guide you to a healthier, happier version of yourself. Here's to tasty meals, better health, and the satisfaction of living a lifestyle that benefits you from the inside out. Cheers to the first step in your transforming journey!

In the following chapters, you'll discover a treasure mine of dishes that not only adhere to The Galveston Diet principles but also appeal to your taste senses, making healthy eating a fun and sustainable part of your daily life.

Beyond the dishes, think of this cookbook as a companion on your holistic wellness journey. The Galveston Diet stresses the interconnectivity of diet, hormones, and lifestyle, empowering you to make informed decisions that meet your body's demands.

Whether you're looking for ideas for a nutritious breakfast, exploring vivid vegetable-based dishes, or appreciating the rich tastes of fish and meats, each recipe is designed with your health and culinary pleasure in mind. You'll realize that fueling your body does not imply compromising taste; rather, it means taking your meals to the next level of delight.

As you read through these pages, remember that this is your journey, and each step is a win. Whether you're a first-time cook or an expert chef, let this cookbook lead you through the process of making not only meals but also moments of well-being.

So let the journey begin! Turn the page, preheat the oven, and prepare to embark on a tasty journey with "The Galveston Diet Cookbook for Beginners." Here's to being healthier, happier, and more tasty!

# Chapter 1: Welcome to The Galveston Diet

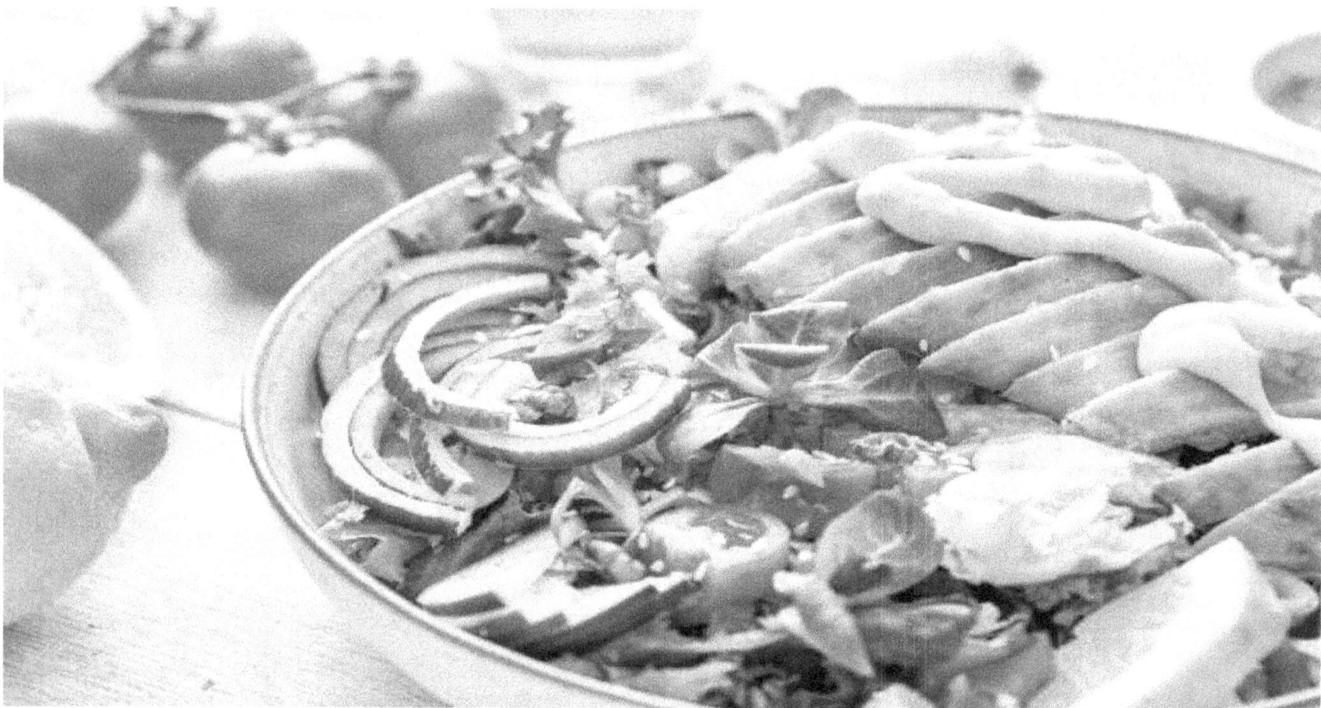

Congratulations and welcome to a transformative culinary journey with "The Galveston Diet Cookbook for Beginners"! In these pages, you are about to embark on a delicious and health-conscious adventure designed to nourish your body while tantalizing your taste buds.

**Embrace a Healthier Lifestyle**

The Galveston Diet isn't just a diet – it's a lifestyle. Developed with the principles of balanced nutrition and mindful eating, this cookbook is your guide to making food choices that support your well-being. It's not about restriction; it's about choosing the right ingredients and flavors that will leave you satisfied and energized.

**Discover the Galveston Flavor**

Galveston cuisine is a celebration of fresh, locally sourced ingredients, and this cookbook brings those flavors to your kitchen. Whether you're a seasoned cook or a novice in the culinary world, the recipes provided will inspire and empower you to create nutritious, mouthwatering meals.

**What to Expect**

Within these pages, you'll find a diverse array of recipes, from wholesome breakfast options to satisfying dinners, and everything in between. Learn about essential tools, explore new ingredients, and master the art of meal planning. The Galveston Diet is not just about eating; it's about embracing a lifestyle that promotes a healthier, happier you.

**Your Personal Wellness Journey**

As you flip through the pages of this cookbook, remember that your wellness journey is unique. Listen to your body, savor each bite, and enjoy the process of creating nourishing meals. Whether you're seeking weight management, increased energy, or simply a renewed love for cooking, The Galveston Diet is here to support you.

# Benefits of The Galveston Diet

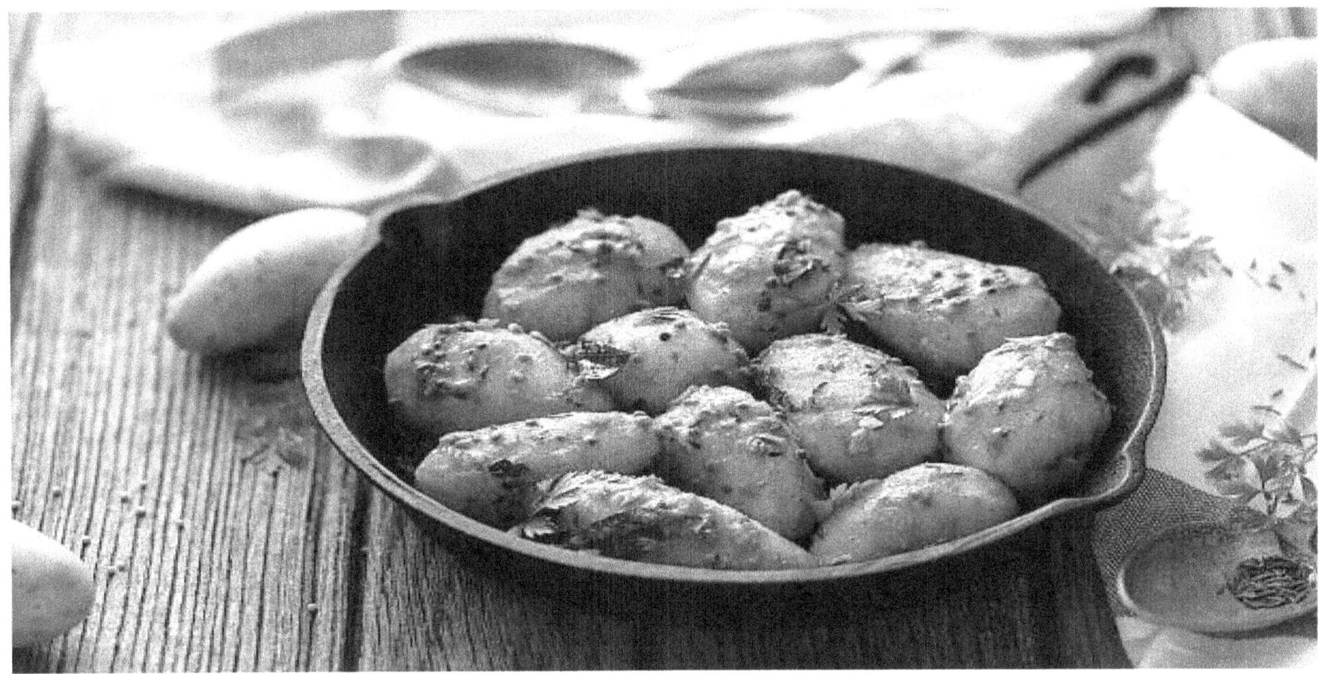

### 1. Balanced Nutrition for Optimal Health

The Galveston Diet places a strong emphasis on balanced nutrition. By incorporating a variety of nutrient-dense foods, you provide your body with the essential vitamins, minerals, and antioxidants it needs. This balance supports overall health, boosts your immune system, and contributes to sustained energy levels throughout the day.

### 2. Weight Management Made Delicious

Say goodbye to restrictive diets and hello to enjoyable, satisfying meals! The Galveston Diet encourages mindful eating and the consumption of wholesome, flavorful foods. By making nutritious choices, you can naturally manage your weight without feeling deprived, fostering a sustainable and healthy relationship with food.

### 3. Inflammation Reduction

Many recipes in The Galveston Diet Cookbook feature ingredients known for their anti-inflammatory properties. By incorporating these elements into your meals, you can potentially reduce inflammation, promoting joint health and overall well-being. Embracing this anti-inflammatory approach may also be beneficial for individuals with specific health concerns.

### 4. Heart-Healthy Choices

The Galveston Diet includes heart-healthy options that focus on promoting cardiovascular well-being. By selecting lean proteins, incorporating omega-3 rich foods, and emphasizing plant-based ingredients, you can support your heart health and reduce the risk of cardiovascular issues.

**5. Enhanced Gut Health**

A healthy gut is the foundation of overall well-being. The Galveston Diet introduces recipes that incorporate fiber-rich foods, probiotics, and prebiotics, promoting a flourishing gut microbiome. A happy gut contributes to improved digestion, nutrient absorption, and even plays a role in supporting mental health.

**6. Sustainable Energy Throughout the Day**

Bid farewell to energy slumps! The Galveston Diet encourages the consumption of nutrient-dense, whole foods that provide a steady release of energy. This sustained energy can enhance focus, productivity, and overall vitality, ensuring you feel your best throughout the day.

**7. Culinary Exploration and Enjoyment**

Discover the joy of cooking and savoring meals that nourish both body and soul. The Galveston Diet Cookbook introduces you to a diverse range of delicious recipes that make healthy eating an exciting and enjoyable experience. Say goodbye to bland and hello to a world of flavors that support your well-being.

# Basics of The Galveston Diet

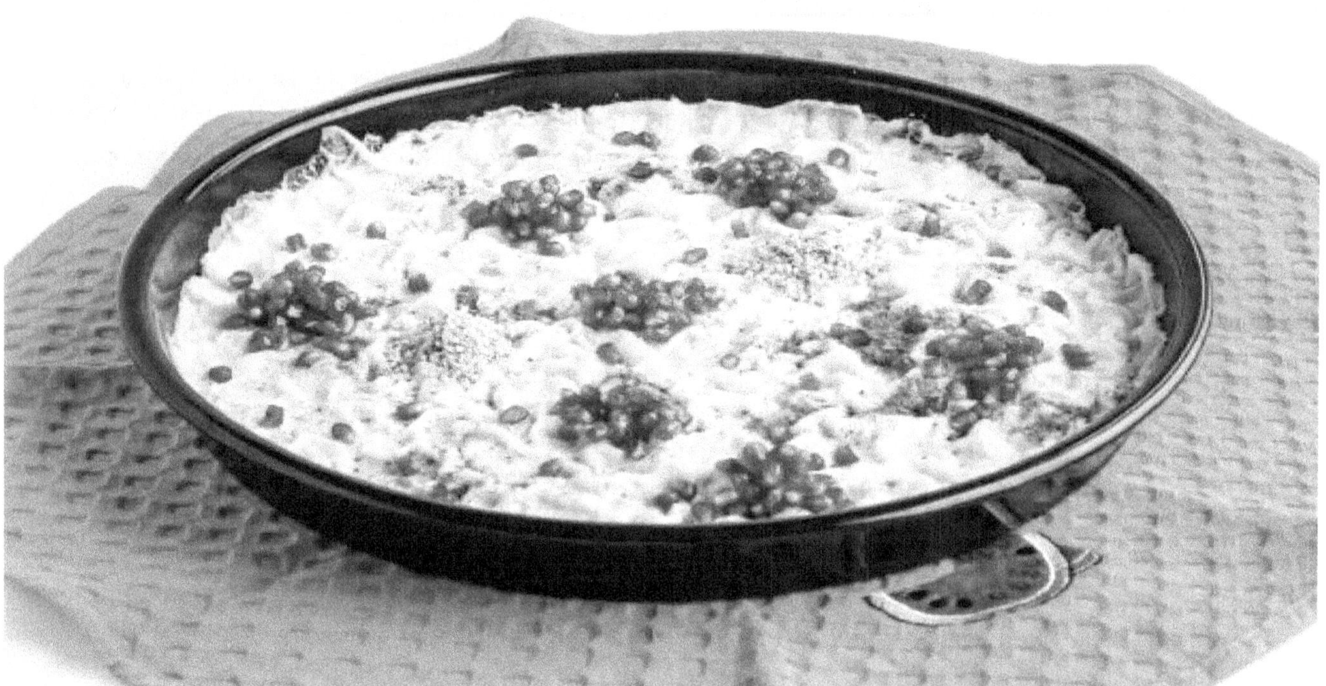

**1. Balanced Macros and Micros**

The Galveston Diet places a strong emphasis on achieving a balance of macronutrients (carbohydrates, proteins, and fats) and micronutrients (vitamins and minerals). By incorporating a variety of whole foods, you ensure that your body receives the essential nutrients it needs for optimal functioning.

## 2. Mindful Eating

Mindful eating is at the heart of The Galveston Diet. Take the time to savor each bite, listen to your body's hunger and fullness cues, and appreciate the flavors and textures of your meals. This mindful approach fosters a healthier relationship with food, helping you make conscious choices that align with your well-being goals.

## 3. Focus on Whole Foods

Say goodbye to highly processed and refined foods! The Galveston Diet encourages the consumption of whole, unprocessed foods. Fresh fruits and vegetables, lean proteins, whole grains, and healthy fats take center stage, providing your body with the nutrients it craves in their most natural and beneficial forms.

## 4. Lean Proteins and Seafood

Proteins are an essential building block for a healthy body, and The Galveston Diet incorporates lean protein sources such as poultry, lean meats, and an emphasis on seafood. Fish, rich in omega-3 fatty acids, not only adds a delightful flavor to your meals but also contributes to heart health and overall well-being.

## 5. Smart Carbohydrate Choices

Carbohydrates play a crucial role in providing energy, and The Galveston Diet encourages smart carbohydrate choices. Opt for whole grains, legumes, and a colorful array of fruits and vegetables to ensure a diverse range of nutrients while maintaining steady energy levels.

## 6. Healthy Fats in Moderation

Embrace the right fats for a balanced diet. The Galveston Diet includes sources of healthy fats, such as avocados, nuts, seeds, and olive oil, which contribute to satiety and support overall health. Moderation is key, ensuring a harmonious balance between all macronutrients.

## 7. Hydration and Detoxification

Staying hydrated is vital for overall health. The Galveston Diet emphasizes the importance of water intake to support proper digestion, nutrient absorption, and detoxification. Infusing water with fresh herbs and fruits adds a burst of flavor while encouraging hydration.

## 8. Individualized Approach

Recognize that every body is unique. The Galveston Diet acknowledges the importance of tailoring dietary choices to individual needs, preferences, and health goals. Listen to your body, adapt recipes to suit your tastes, and enjoy the flexibility of this approach.

# Getting Started with The Galveston Diet

## 1. Educate Yourself

Before diving into the kitchen, take a moment to understand the core principles of The Galveston Diet. Familiarize yourself with the emphasis on balanced nutrition, whole foods, and the benefits of lean proteins, healthy fats, and smart carbohydrates. The more you know, the more confident and informed your choices will be.

## 2. Assess Your Goals

Define your health and wellness goals. Whether you're looking to manage your weight, boost energy levels, or improve overall well-being, having clear objectives will help tailor The Galveston Diet to your specific needs. Remember, each person's journey is unique, so your goals are personal to you.

## 3. Kitchen Preparation

Set yourself up for success by organizing your kitchen. Stock up on essential tools, including quality knives, cutting boards, and cookware. Ensure your pantry is well-stocked with staples such as whole grains, herbs, spices, and healthy oils. Having a well-prepared kitchen makes meal preparation enjoyable and efficient.

## 4. Understand Portion Control

While The Galveston Diet focuses on nourishing your body with wholesome foods, portion control remains a key aspect. Be mindful of serving sizes to maintain a balanced and sustainable approach. Learning to listen to your body's hunger and fullness cues will help you make informed choices during meals.

## 5. Meal Planning

Plan your meals ahead of time to streamline your journey. Create a weekly meal plan that incorporates a variety of flavors and nutrients. This not only saves you time but also ensures you have the necessary ingredients on hand, reducing the temptation to opt for less healthy alternatives.

## 6. Explore New Ingredients

Open your palate to a world of fresh, seasonal ingredients. The Galveston Diet encourages culinary exploration, so don't be afraid to try new fruits, vegetables, and whole grains. Experimenting with a diverse range of ingredients adds excitement to your meals and broadens your nutritional intake.

## 7. Stay Hydrated

Hydration is a fundamental aspect of The Galveston Diet. Water supports digestion, aids in detoxification, and keeps your body functioning optimally. Make a habit of drinking enough water throughout the day, and consider infusing it with herbs or citrus for added flavor.

## 8. Listen to Your Body

Remember that The Galveston Diet is a journey, not a destination. Listen to your body's signals, adapt recipes to suit your tastes, and be flexible in your approach. If you're unsure about certain foods or have specific dietary concerns, consult with a healthcare professional for personalized advice.

# Understanding The Galveston Diet Principles

## 1. Balanced Nutrition

At the heart of The Galveston Diet is the concept of balanced nutrition. This means incorporating a variety of nutrient-dense foods to ensure your body receives the essential vitamins, minerals, and macronutrients it needs for optimal functioning. Embrace a colorful array of fruits, vegetables, lean proteins, whole grains, and healthy fats to create meals that are both delicious and nutritionally robust.

## 2. Mindful Eating

Mindful eating is a cornerstone of The Galveston Diet. Slow down, savor each bite, and pay attention to your body's hunger and fullness cues. By being present during meals, you can develop a healthier relationship with food, making it easier to make conscious choices that align with your well-being goals.

## 3. Whole, Unprocessed Foods

Bid farewell to highly processed and refined foods. The Galveston Diet encourages the consumption of whole, unprocessed foods that retain their natural goodness. Fresh fruits and vegetables, lean proteins, whole grains, and healthy fats take center stage, providing a diverse range of nutrients without unnecessary additives or preservatives.

## 4. Lean Proteins and Seafood Emphasis

Proteins are essential for building and repairing tissues, and The Galveston Diet places a particular emphasis on lean protein sources. Incorporating poultry, lean meats, and seafood not only adds delicious flavors to your meals but also provides essential amino acids. Seafood, rich in omega-3 fatty acids, further contributes to heart health and overall well-being.

## 5. Smart Carbohydrate Choices

Carbohydrates are a vital energy source, and The Galveston Diet encourages smart carbohydrate choices. Opt for whole grains, legumes, and a rainbow of fruits and vegetables to ensure a diverse range of nutrients. This approach maintains steady energy levels while providing your body with essential fiber and antioxidants.

## 6. Healthy Fats in Moderation

Embrace the right fats for a balanced diet. The Galveston Diet includes sources of healthy fats, such as avocados, nuts, seeds, and olive oil. While these fats are beneficial, moderation is key to maintaining a healthy balance between all macronutrients.

## 7. Hydration for Wellness

Water is an essential component of The Galveston Diet. Staying adequately hydrated supports digestion, nutrient absorption, and detoxification. Make a habit of drinking water throughout the day and consider infusing it with fresh herbs or fruits to add a burst of flavor.

**8. Individualized Approach**

Recognize that everyone is unique, and The Galveston Diet acknowledges the importance of tailoring dietary choices to individual needs, preferences, and health goals. Listen to your body, adapt recipes to suit your tastes, and enjoy the flexibility of this approach.

# Chapter 2: Breakfast



**Prep Time:** 10 minutes
**Cook Time:** 0 minutes
**Serving Size:** 1

**Ingredients:**

- 1 cup spinach leaves

- 1/2 banana, frozen

- 1/2 cup Greek yogurt

- 1/4 cup blueberries

- 1 tablespoon chia seeds

- 1 tablespoon almond butter

- 1/2 cup almond milk

**Instructions:**

1. Blend spinach, banana, Greek yogurt, blueberries, chia seeds, almond butter, and almond milk until smooth.

2. Pour into a bowl and top with additional blueberries and a sprinkle of chia seeds.

**Nutritional Information:**

- Calories: 350

- Protein: 15g

- Fat: 18g

- Carbohydrates: 40g

- Fiber: 10g

# Avocado and Smoked Salmon Toast

**Prep Time:** 15 minutes

**Cook Time:** 5 minutes

**Serving Size:** 2

## Ingredients:

- 2 slices whole-grain bread

- 1 ripe avocado

- 4 oz smoked salmon

- 1 tablespoon capers

- 1 tablespoon chopped dill

- Lemon wedges for serving

## Instructions:

1. Toast the whole-grain bread slices to your liking.

2. Mash the ripe avocado and spread it evenly on the toasted bread.

3. Top with smoked salmon, capers, and chopped dill.

4. Serve with lemon wedges on the side.

## Nutritional Information:

- Calories: 320

- Protein: 20g

- Fat: 18g

- Carbohydrates: 25g

- Fiber: 10g

**Prep Time:** 5 minutes

**Cook Time:** 15 minutes

**Serving Size:** 2

**Ingredients:**

- 1 cup cooked quinoa

- 1/2 cup mixed berries (strawberries, blueberries, raspberries)

- 2 tablespoons Greek yogurt

- 1 tablespoon honey

- 1/4 cup sliced almonds

**Instructions:**

1. In a bowl, layer cooked quinoa, mixed berries, and Greek yogurt.

2. Drizzle honey over the top and sprinkle with sliced almonds.

**Nutritional Information:**

- Calories: 280

- Protein: 8g

- Fat: 10g

- Carbohydrates: 40g

- Fiber: 6g

# Egg and Veggie Breakfast Wrap

**Prep Time:** 10 minutes

**Cook Time:** 5 minutes

**Serving Size:** 1

**Ingredients:**

- 1 whole-grain tortilla
- 2 eggs, scrambled
- 1/4 cup diced bell peppers
- 1/4 cup diced tomatoes
- 2 tablespoons feta cheese
- Fresh cilantro for garnish

**Instructions:**

1. In a skillet, scramble the eggs until cooked through.
2. Warm the whole-grain tortilla.
3. Fill the tortilla with scrambled eggs, diced bell peppers, diced tomatoes, and feta cheese.
4. Garnish with fresh cilantro.

**Nutritional Information:**

- Calories: 320
- Protein: 18g
- Fat: 15g
- Carbohydrates: 28g
- Fiber: 5g

**Prep Time:** 5 minutes (plus overnight chilling)
**Cook Time:** 0 minutes
**Serving Size:** 1

**Ingredients:**

- 2 tablespoons chia seeds

- 1/2 cup almond milk

- 1/2 teaspoon vanilla extract

- 1/4 cup granola

- 1/4 cup mixed berries

**Instructions:**

1. In a jar, mix chia seeds, almond milk, and vanilla extract. Refrigerate overnight.

2. In the morning, layer chia seed pudding with granola and mixed berries in a glass.

**Nutritional Information:**

- Calories: 220

- Protein: 6g

- Fat: 10g

- Carbohydrates: 30g

- Fiber: 8g

# Sweet Potato and Black Bean Breakfast Hash

**Prep Time:** 15 minutes

**Cook Time:** 20 minutes

**Serving Size:** 2

**Ingredients:**

- 1 large sweet potato, diced

- 1 can (15 oz) black beans, drained and rinsed

- 1 bell pepper, diced

- 1/2 red onion, diced

- 2 eggs

- 1 tablespoon olive oil

- Salt and pepper to taste

- Fresh cilantro for garnish

**Instructions:**

1. In a skillet, heat olive oil and sauté sweet potatoes until slightly tender.

2. Add black beans, bell pepper, and red onion. Cook until vegetables are cooked through.

3. Create wells in the hash and crack eggs into them. Cover and cook until eggs are done to your liking.

4. Season with salt and pepper, garnish with fresh cilantro, and serve.

**Nutritional Information:**

- Calories: 380

- Protein: 16g

- Fat: 12g

- Carbohydrates: 55g

- Fiber: 15g

Blueberry Almond Overnight Oats

# Blueberry Almond Overnight Oats

**Prep Time:** 5 minutes (plus overnight chilling)
**Cook Time:** 0 minutes
**Serving Size:** 1

**Ingredients:**

- 1/2 cup rolled oats
- 1/2 cup almond milk
- 1/4 cup Greek yogurt
- 1/4 cup blueberries
- 1 tablespoon almond butter
- 1 tablespoon honey

**Instructions:**

1. In a jar, combine rolled oats, almond milk, Greek yogurt, blueberries, almond butter, and honey. Stir well.
2. Refrigerate overnight.
3. In the morning, give it a good stir and enjoy.

**Nutritional Information:**

- Calories: 280
- Protein: 12g
- Fat: 10g
- Carbohydrates: 40g
- Fiber: 7g

Spinach and Mushroom Omelette

# Spinach and Mushroom Omelette

**Prep Time:** 10 minutes

**Cook Time:** 5 minutes

**Serving Size:** 1

**Ingredients:**

- 2 eggs, beaten
- 1 cup fresh spinach
- 1/2 cup sliced mushrooms
- 1/4 cup feta cheese
- Salt and pepper to taste
- 1 teaspoon olive oil

**Instructions:**

1. In a skillet, sauté spinach and mushrooms in olive oil until wilted.
2. Pour beaten eggs over the vegetables and cook until set.
3. Sprinkle feta cheese over one half of the omelette, fold, and serve.

**Nutritional Information:**

- Calories: 300
- Protein: 20g
- Fat: 22g
- Carbohydrates: 5g
- Fiber: 2g

# Coconut Mango Chia Pudding

**Prep Time:** 10 minutes (plus chilling)
**Cook Time:** 0 minutes
**Serving Size:** 2

**Ingredients:**

- 4 tablespoons chia seeds

- 1 cup coconut milk

- 1 teaspoon vanilla extract

- 1 ripe mango, diced

- Shredded coconut for garnish

**Instructions:**

1. In a bowl, mix chia seeds, coconut milk, and vanilla extract. Refrigerate for at least 2 hours or overnight.

2. Layer chia pudding with diced mango in serving glasses.

3. Garnish with shredded coconut before serving.

**Nutritional Information:**

- Calories: 250

- Protein: 5g

- Fat: 20g

- Carbohydrates: 20g

- Fiber: 8g

Coconut Mango Chia Pudding

# Peanut Butter Banana Protein Pancakes

**Prep Time:** 15 minutes

**Cook Time:** 10 minutes

**Serving Size:** 2

**Ingredients:**

- 1 cup whole wheat flour

- 1 scoop vanilla protein powder

- 1 teaspoon baking powder

- 1/2 teaspoon cinnamon

- 1 ripe banana, mashed

- 2 eggs

- 1 cup almond milk

- 2 tablespoons peanut butter (plus extra for topping)

**Instructions:**

1. In a bowl, mix whole wheat flour, protein powder, baking powder, and cinnamon.

2. In a separate bowl, whisk together mashed banana, eggs, almond milk, and peanut butter.

3. Combine wet and dry ingredients until just mixed.

4. Cook pancakes on a griddle or skillet until golden brown on both sides.

5. Serve with a drizzle of peanut butter on top.

**Nutritional Information:**

- Calories: 400

- Protein: 25g

- Fat: 15g

- Carbohydrates: 45g

- Fiber: 8g

**Prep Time:** 10 minutes

**Cook Time:** 10 minutes

**Serving Size:** 1

**Ingredients:**

- 2 whole-grain tortillas

- 1 cup fresh spinach

- 1/2 cup sliced mushrooms

- 1/4 cup shredded mozzarella cheese

- 1/4 teaspoon garlic powder

- Salsa for serving

**Instructions:**

1. In a skillet, sauté spinach and mushrooms until wilted.

2. Place one tortilla in the skillet, add the sautéed vegetables, sprinkle with mozzarella cheese, and top with the second tortilla.

3. Cook until the cheese is melted and the tortillas are golden brown.

4. Slice into wedges and serve with salsa.

**Nutritional Information:**

- Calories: 320

- Protein: 15g

- Fat: 12g

- Carbohydrates: 40g

- Fiber: 8g

# Banana Nut Quinoa Porridge

**Prep Time:** 5 minutes

**Cook Time:** 15 minutes

**Serving Size:** 1

**Ingredients:**

- 1/2 cup cooked quinoa

- 1/2 cup almond milk

- 1 ripe banana, mashed

- 1 tablespoon chopped walnuts

- 1/2 teaspoon cinnamon

- Drizzle of honey

**Instructions:**

1. In a saucepan, combine cooked quinoa, almond milk, mashed banana, chopped walnuts, and cinnamon.

2. Heat over medium heat until warmed through.

3. Drizzle with honey before serving.

**Nutritional Information:**

- Calories: 280

- Protein: 8g

- Fat: 12g

- Carbohydrates: 40g

- Fiber: 6g

# Turmeric and Kale Breakfast Scramble

**Prep Time:** 10 minutes
**Cook Time:** 10 minutes
**Serving Size:** 2

**Ingredients:**

- 4 eggs, beaten

- 1 cup chopped kale

- 1/2 teaspoon turmeric powder

- 1/4 teaspoon cumin

- Salt and pepper to taste

- 1 tablespoon olive oil

- Cherry tomatoes for garnish

**Instructions:**

1. In a skillet, sauté chopped kale in olive oil until slightly wilted.

2. Add beaten eggs, turmeric powder, cumin, salt, and pepper. Scramble until eggs are cooked.

3. Garnish with cherry tomatoes before serving.

**Nutritional Information:**

- Calories: 320

- Protein: 20g

- Fat: 22g

- Carbohydrates: 8g

- Fiber: 2g

# Pineapple Coconut Chia Smoothie

**Prep Time:** 5 minutes

**Cook Time:** 0 minutes

**Serving Size:** 1

**Ingredients:**

- 1 cup coconut water

- 1/2 cup pineapple chunks

- 1/4 cup chia seeds

- 1/4 cup shredded coconut

- 1 tablespoon lime juice

**Instructions:**

1. In a blender, combine coconut water, pineapple chunks, chia seeds, shredded coconut, and lime juice.

2. Blend until smooth.

3. Pour into a glass and enjoy.

**Nutritional Information:**

- Calories: 250

- Protein: 6g

- Fat: 12g

- Carbohydrates: 30g

- Fiber: 10g

Pineapple Coconut Chia Smoothie

**Prep Time:** 10 minutes

**Cook Time:** 0 minutes

**Serving Size:** 1

**Ingredients:**

- 1 cup low-fat cottage cheese

- 1/2 cup mixed berries (strawberries, blueberries, raspberries)

- 1/4 cup granola

- 1 tablespoon honey

**Instructions:**

1. In a glass, layer low-fat cottage cheese with mixed berries and granola.

2. Drizzle with honey before serving.

**Nutritional Information:**

- Calories: 280

- Protein: 18g

- Fat: 8g

- Carbohydrates: 35g

- Fiber: 5g

# Chapter 3: Snacks and appetizers

## Greek Yogurt and Veggie Dip

**Prep Time:** 10 minutes

**Cook Time:** 0 minutes

**Serving Size:** 4

**Ingredients:**

- 1 cup Greek yogurt

- 1/2 cucumber, finely diced

- 1/2 red bell pepper, finely diced

- 1 tablespoon fresh dill, chopped

- 1 clove garlic, minced

- Salt and pepper to taste

- Whole-grain pita chips for serving

**Instructions:**

1. In a bowl, combine Greek yogurt, cucumber, red bell pepper, dill, and minced garlic.

2. Season with salt and pepper to taste.

3. Chill in the refrigerator for at least 30 minutes.

4. Serve with whole-grain pita chips.

**Nutritional Information:**

- Calories: 120

- Protein: 8g

- Fat: 2g

- Carbohydrates: 18g

- Fiber: 3g

# Avocado and Tomato Salsa

**Prep Time:** 15 minutes

**Cook Time:** 0 minutes

**Serving Size:** 6

**Ingredients:**

- 2 avocados, diced

- 1 cup cherry tomatoes, quartered

- 1/4 red onion, finely diced

- 1/4 cup cilantro, chopped

- 1 jalapeño, seeded and minced

- Juice of 1 lime

- Salt and pepper to taste

- Whole-grain tortilla chips for serving

**Instructions:**

1. In a bowl, gently mix together diced avocados, cherry tomatoes, red onion, cilantro, jalapeño, and lime juice.

2. Season with salt and pepper to taste.

3. Allow flavors to meld in the refrigerator for 15 minutes.

4. Serve with whole-grain tortilla chips.

**Nutritional Information:**

- Calories: 160

- Protein: 2g

- Fat: 12g

- Carbohydrates: 15g

- Fiber: 6g

**Prep Time:** 20 minutes
**Cook Time:** 25 minutes
**Serving Size:** 4

**Ingredients:**

- 1 cup cooked quinoa

- 1 can (15 oz) black beans, drained and rinsed

- 1 cup corn kernels (fresh or frozen)

- 1 cup cherry tomatoes, halved

- 1/4 cup red onion, finely diced

- 1 teaspoon cumin

- 1 teaspoon chili powder

- Salt and pepper to taste

- Mini bell peppers, halved and seeds removed

**Instructions:**

1. In a bowl, mix together cooked quinoa, black beans, corn, cherry tomatoes, red onion, cumin, chili powder, salt, and pepper.

2. Stuff mini bell peppers with the quinoa mixture.

3. Bake in a preheated oven at 375°F (190°C) for 25 minutes.

4. Serve warm.

**Nutritional Information:**

- Calories: 220

- Protein: 8g

- Fat: 2g

- Carbohydrates: 45g

- Fiber: 8g

# Cucumber and Hummus Bites

**Prep Time:** 10 minutes

**Cook Time:** 0 minutes

**Serving Size:** 4

**Ingredients:**

- 2 large cucumbers, sliced into rounds

- 1/2 cup hummus

- Cherry tomatoes, halved

- Fresh parsley for garnish

**Instructions:**

1. Arrange cucumber slices on a serving platter.

2. Spoon a dollop of hummus onto each cucumber slice.

3. Top with a halved cherry tomato and garnish with fresh parsley.

**Nutritional Information:**

- Calories: 80

- Protein: 3g

- Fat: 4g

- Carbohydrates: 10g

- Fiber: 3g

**Prep Time:** 25 minutes

**Cook Time:** 0 minutes

**Serving Size:** 6

**Ingredients:**

- 6 rice paper wrappers

- 1 ripe mango, thinly sliced

- 1 avocado, thinly sliced

- 1 cucumber, julienned

- 1 cup mixed greens

- Fresh mint leaves

- Sweet chili sauce for dipping

**Instructions:**

1. Dip rice paper wrappers in warm water for a few seconds until pliable.

2. Lay each wrapper flat and fill with mango slices, avocado slices, julienned cucumber, mixed greens, and mint leaves.

3. Fold in the sides and roll tightly.

4. Serve with sweet chili sauce for dipping.

**Nutritional Information:**

- Calories: 150

- Protein: 2g

- Fat: 5g

- Carbohydrates: 25g

- Fiber: 4g

# Baked Sweet Potato Fries with Greek Yogurt Dip

**Prep Time:** 15 minutes

**Cook Time:** 25 minutes

**Serving Size:** 4

**Ingredients:**

- 2 large sweet potatoes, cut into fries
- 2 tablespoons olive oil
- 1 teaspoon paprika
- 1 teaspoon garlic powder
- Salt and pepper to taste
- 1 cup Greek yogurt
- 1 tablespoon lemon juice
- Fresh chives for garnish

**Instructions:**

1. Preheat the oven to 425°F (220°C).
2. Toss sweet potato fries with olive oil, paprika, garlic powder, salt, and pepper.
3. Spread fries on a baking sheet and bake for 25 minutes or until golden and crispy.
4. In a bowl, mix Greek yogurt with lemon juice.
5. Garnish sweet potato fries with fresh chives and serve with the Greek yogurt dip.

**Nutritional Information:**

- Calories: 250
- Protein: 8g
- Fat: 8g
- Carbohydrates: 40g
- Fiber: 6g

Baked Sweet Potato Fries with Greek Yogurt Dip

# Edamame and Sea Salt Snack

**Prep Time:** 5 minutes
**Cook Time:** 5 minutes
**Serving Size:** 2

**Ingredients:**

- 2 cups edamame, steamed

- Sea salt to taste

**Instructions:**

1. Steam edamame according to package instructions.

2. Sprinkle with sea salt while still warm.

3. Toss to coat evenly.

4. Serve as a nutritious and protein-packed snack.

**Nutritional Information:**

- Calories: 150

- Protein: 13g

- Fat: 6g

- Carbohydrates: 12g

- Fiber: 8g

# Caprese Skewers with Balsamic Glaze

**Prep Time:** 15 minutes
**Cook Time:** 0 minutes
**Serving Size:** 4

**Ingredients:**

- Cherry tomatoes
- Fresh mozzarella balls
- Fresh basil leaves
- Balsamic glaze for drizzling
- Wooden skewers

**Instructions:**

1. Thread a cherry tomato, a mozzarella ball, and a fresh basil leaf onto each skewer.
2. Arrange skewers on a serving platter.
3. Drizzle with balsamic glaze just before serving.

**Nutritional Information:**

- Calories: 120
- Protein: 6g
- Fat: 8g
- Carbohydrates: 6g
- Fiber: 2g

Caprese Skewers with Balsamic Glaze

# Spicy Roasted Chickpeas

**Prep Time:** 10 minutes
**Cook Time:** 30 minutes
**Serving Size:** 4

**Ingredients:**

- 2 cans (15 oz each) chickpeas, drained and rinsed

- 2 tablespoons olive oil

- 1 teaspoon smoked paprika

- 1/2 teaspoon cayenne pepper

- 1/2 teaspoon garlic powder

- Salt to taste

**Instructions:**

1. Preheat the oven to 400°F (200°C).

2. In a bowl, toss chickpeas with olive oil, smoked paprika, cayenne pepper, garlic powder, and salt.

3. Spread chickpeas on a baking sheet and roast for 30 minutes or until crispy.

4. Allow to cool before serving.

**Nutritional Information:**

- Calories: 180

- Protein: 8g

- Fat: 8g

- Carbohydrates: 20g

- Fiber: 5g

# Stuffed Jalapeños with Turkey and Cream Cheese

**Prep Time:** 20 minutes

**Cook Time:** 15 minutes

**Serving Size:** 4

**Ingredients:**

- 8 large jalapeños, halved and seeds removed

- 1/2 lb ground turkey

- 1/4 cup red onion, finely diced

- 2 cloves garlic, minced

- 4 oz cream cheese, softened

- 1 teaspoon cumin

- 1/2 teaspoon chili powder

- Salt and pepper to taste

- Fresh cilantro for garnish

**Instructions:**

1. Preheat the oven to 375°F (190°C).

2. In a skillet, cook ground turkey until browned. Add red onion and garlic, cooking until softened.

3. In a bowl, mix cooked turkey, cream cheese, cumin, chili powder, salt, and pepper.

4. Stuff jalapeño halves with the turkey mixture.

5. Bake for 15 minutes or until jalapeños are tender.

6. Garnish with fresh cilantro before serving.

**Nutritional Information:**

- Calories: 220

- Protein: 15g

- Fat: 12g

- Carbohydrates: 15g

- Fiber: 3g

## Zucchini Noodle Bruschetta

**Prep Time:** 15 minutes
**Cook Time:** 0 minutes
**Serving Size:** 4

**Ingredients:**

- 2 large zucchinis, spiralized into noodles

- 1 cup cherry tomatoes, diced

- 1/4 cup red onion, finely chopped

- 2 cloves garlic, minced

- 2 tablespoons balsamic vinegar

- 1 tablespoon olive oil

- Fresh basil for garnish

- Salt and pepper to taste

**Instructions:**

1. In a bowl, combine zucchini noodles, cherry tomatoes, red onion, and minced garlic.

2. Drizzle with balsamic vinegar and olive oil, tossing gently.

3. Season with salt and pepper.

4. Garnish with fresh basil before serving.

**Nutritional Information:**

- Calories: 90

- Protein: 3g

- Fat: 5g

- Carbohydrates: 10g

- Fiber: 3g

# Smoked Salmon Cucumber Bites

**Prep Time:** 10 minutes

**Cook Time:** 0 minutes

**Serving Size:** 6

**Ingredients:**

- 1 English cucumber, sliced into rounds

- 4 oz smoked salmon

- 1/4 cup cream cheese

- Fresh dill for garnish

- Lemon zest for topping

**Instructions:**

1. Arrange cucumber rounds on a serving platter.

2. Spread a thin layer of cream cheese on each cucumber round.

3. Top with smoked salmon.

4. Garnish with fresh dill and a sprinkle of lemon zest.

**Nutritional Information:**

- Calories: 70

- Protein: 5g

- Fat: 5g

- Carbohydrates: 2g

- Fiber: 0g

Turmeric Roasted Chickpea Snack Mix

**Prep Time:** 10 minutes

**Cook Time:** 30 minutes

**Serving Size:** 8

**Ingredients:**

- 2 cans (15 oz each) chickpeas, drained and rinsed

- 2 tablespoons olive oil

- 1 teaspoon turmeric

- 1/2 teaspoon cumin

- 1/2 teaspoon smoked paprika

- 1/4 teaspoon cayenne pepper

- 1 cup mixed nuts

- 1 cup whole-grain pretzels

**Instructions:**

1. Preheat the oven to 400°F (200°C).

2. In a bowl, toss chickpeas and mixed nuts with olive oil, turmeric, cumin, smoked paprika, and cayenne pepper.

3. Spread on a baking sheet and bake for 30 minutes or until golden and crispy.

4. Mix in whole-grain pretzels and let cool before serving.

**Nutritional Information:**

- Calories: 180

- Protein: 7g

- Fat: 10g

- Carbohydrates: 18g

- Fiber: 4g

Turmeric Roasted Chickpea Snack Mix

# Cauliflower Buffalo Bites

**Prep Time:** 15 minutes

**Cook Time:** 25 minutes

**Serving Size:** 4

**Ingredients:**

- 1 head cauliflower, cut into florets

- 1/2 cup whole wheat flour

- 1/2 cup water

- 1 teaspoon garlic powder

- 1 teaspoon onion powder

- 1/2 teaspoon smoked paprika

- Salt and pepper to taste

- 1/2 cup buffalo sauce

- Greek yogurt for dipping

**Instructions:**

1. Preheat the oven to 425°F (220°C).

2. In a bowl, whisk together whole wheat flour, water, garlic powder, onion powder, smoked paprika, salt, and pepper.

3. Dip cauliflower florets into the batter and place on a baking sheet.

4. Bake for 25 minutes or until crispy.

5. Toss with buffalo sauce before serving and serve with Greek yogurt for dipping.

**Nutritional Information:**

- Calories: 120

- Protein: 5g

- Fat: 2g

- Carbohydrates: 20g

- Fiber: 5g

# Mediterranean Stuffed Mushrooms

**Prep Time:** 20 minutes
**Cook Time:** 15 minutes
**Serving Size:** 4

**Ingredients:**

- 16 large button mushrooms, stems removed

- 1/2 cup quinoa, cooked

- 1/4 cup Kalamata olives, chopped

- 1/4 cup sun-dried tomatoes, chopped

- 1/4 cup feta cheese, crumbled

- 2 tablespoons fresh parsley, chopped

- 1 clove garlic, minced

- 1 tablespoon olive oil

- Salt and pepper to taste

**Instructions:**

1. Preheat the oven to 375°F (190°C).

2. In a bowl, mix together quinoa, Kalamata olives, sun-dried tomatoes, feta cheese, parsley, minced garlic, olive oil, salt, and pepper.

3. Stuff each mushroom with the quinoa mixture.

4. Bake for 15 minutes or until mushrooms are tender.

5. Serve warm.

**Nutritional Information:**

- Calories: 140

- Protein: 6g

- Fat: 7g

- Carbohydrates: 15g

- Fiber: 3g

# Chapter 4: Vegetables and sides

## Roasted Brussels Sprouts with Balsamic Glaze

**Prep Time:** 10 minutes
**Cook Time:** 25 minutes
**Serving Size:** 4

**Ingredients:**

- 1 lb Brussels sprouts, trimmed and halved

- 2 tablespoons olive oil

- Salt and pepper to taste

- 2 tablespoons balsamic glaze

**Instructions:**

1. Preheat the oven to 400°F (200°C).

2. Toss Brussels sprouts with olive oil, salt, and pepper.

3. Spread on a baking sheet and roast for 25 minutes or until golden.

4. Drizzle with balsamic glaze before serving.

**Nutritional Information:**

- Calories: 120

- Protein: 5g

- Fat: 7g

- Carbohydrates: 15g

- Fiber: 6g

# Quinoa and Vegetable Stir-Fry

**Prep Time:** 15 minutes
**Cook Time:** 20 minutes
**Serving Size:** 6

**Ingredients:**

- 1 cup quinoa, cooked

- 1 tablespoon sesame oil

- 1 cup broccoli florets

- 1 bell pepper, thinly sliced

- 1 carrot, julienned

- 1 zucchini, sliced

- 3 green onions, chopped

- 2 tablespoons low-sodium soy sauce

- 1 tablespoon rice vinegar

- 1 teaspoon ginger, grated

**Instructions:**

1. In a wok or skillet, heat sesame oil over medium heat.

2. Stir-fry broccoli, bell pepper, carrot, and zucchini until tender-crisp.

3. Add cooked quinoa and green onions to the vegetables.

4. In a small bowl, mix soy sauce, rice vinegar, and ginger. Pour over the quinoa and vegetables.

5. Toss until well combined and serve hot.

**Nutritional Information:**

- Calories: 180

- Protein: 8g

- Fat: 4g

- Carbohydrates: 30g

- Fiber: 5g

## Garlic Roasted Asparagus

**Prep Time:** 5 minutes
**Cook Time:** 12 minutes
**Serving Size:** 4

**Ingredients:**

- 1 lb asparagus, trimmed

- 2 tablespoons olive oil

- 3 cloves garlic, minced

- Salt and pepper to taste

- Lemon wedges for serving

**Instructions:**

1. Preheat the oven to 425°F (220°C).

2. Toss asparagus with olive oil, minced garlic, salt, and pepper.

3. Spread on a baking sheet and roast for 12 minutes or until tender.

4. Squeeze lemon wedges over the roasted asparagus before serving.

**Nutritional Information:**

- Calories: 90

- Protein: 4g

- Fat: 7g

- Carbohydrates: 7g

- Fiber: 4g

# Cauliflower and Chickpea Curry

**Prep Time:** 15 minutes
**Cook Time:** 25 minutes
**Serving Size:** 4

**Ingredients:**

- 1 head cauliflower, cut into florets
- 1 can (15 oz) chickpeas, drained and rinsed
- 1 onion, finely chopped
- 2 cloves garlic, minced
- 1 can (14 oz) diced tomatoes
- 1 can (14 oz) coconut milk
- 2 tablespoons curry powder
- 1 teaspoon turmeric
- Salt and pepper to taste
- Fresh cilantro for garnish

**Instructions:**

1. In a large pot, sauté onion and garlic until softened.
2. Add cauliflower, chickpeas, diced tomatoes, coconut milk, curry powder, turmeric, salt, and pepper.
3. Simmer for 20-25 minutes or until cauliflower is tender.
4. Garnish with fresh cilantro before serving.

**Nutritional Information:**

- Calories: 280
- Protein: 10g
- Fat: 15g
- Carbohydrates: 30g
- Fiber: 8g

# Spaghetti Squash Primavera

**Prep Time:** 15 minutes

**Cook Time:** 45 minutes

**Serving Size:** 4

**Ingredients:**

- 1 medium spaghetti squash

- 2 tablespoons olive oil

- 1 bell pepper, thinly sliced

- 1 zucchini, thinly sliced

- 1 carrot, julienned

- 2 cloves garlic, minced

- 1 cup cherry tomatoes, halved

- 1/4 cup fresh basil, chopped

- Salt and pepper to taste

**Instructions:**

1. Preheat the oven to 400°F (200°C).

2. Cut the spaghetti squash in half lengthwise and scoop out the seeds.

3. Drizzle with olive oil, season with salt and pepper, and place cut-side down on a baking sheet.

4. Roast for 45 minutes or until the squash is tender.

5. In a skillet, sauté bell pepper, zucchini, carrot, and garlic until tender.

6. Scrape the spaghetti squash into strands using a fork and toss with the sautéed vegetables.

7. Add cherry tomatoes and fresh basil. Toss gently and serve.

**Nutritional Information:**

- Calories: 150

- Protein: 3g

- Fat: 8g

- Carbohydrates: 20g

- Fiber: 5g

## Lemon Garlic Roasted Broccoli

**Prep Time:** 10 minutes
**Cook Time:** 20 minutes
**Serving Size:** 4

**Ingredients:**

- 1 lb broccoli florets

- 2 tablespoons olive oil

- 2 cloves garlic, minced

- Zest of 1 lemon

- Salt and pepper to taste

**Instructions:**

1. Preheat the oven to 425°F (220°C).

2. Toss broccoli with olive oil, minced garlic, lemon zest, salt, and pepper.

3. Spread on a baking sheet and roast for 20 minutes or until edges are golden.

4. Serve hot.

**Nutritional Information:**

- Calories: 90

- Protein: 5g

- Fat: 6g

- Carbohydrates: 8g

- Fiber: 4g

**Prep Time:** 20 minutes

**Cook Time:** 20 minutes

**Serving Size:** 6

**Ingredients:**

- 2 cups sweet potatoes, grated

- 1 cup quinoa, cooked

- 1/2 cup whole wheat breadcrumbs

- 1/4 cup red onion, finely chopped

- 1 teaspoon cumin

- 1 teaspoon paprika

- Salt and pepper to taste

- Greek yogurt for dipping

**Instructions:**

1. In a bowl, mix together grated sweet potatoes, cooked quinoa, breadcrumbs, red onion, cumin, paprika, salt, and pepper.

2. Form the mixture into patties.

3. Heat a skillet over medium heat and cook patties for 4-5 minutes per side or until golden brown.

4. Serve with a dollop of Greek yogurt on top.

**Nutritional Information:**

- Calories: 180

- Protein: 6g

- Fat: 2g

- Carbohydrates: 35g

- Fiber: 5g

Sweet Potato and Quinoa Patties

# Green Bean Almondine

**Prep Time:** 10 minutes

**Cook Time:** 10 minutes

**Serving Size:** 4

**Ingredients:**

- 1 lb green beans, trimmed
- 2 tablespoons olive oil
- 1/4 cup almonds, sliced
- 2 cloves garlic, minced
- Juice of 1 lemon
- Salt and pepper to taste

**Instructions:**

1. Blanch green beans in boiling water for 3-4 minutes. Drain and set aside.
2. In a skillet, heat olive oil over medium heat.
3. Add sliced almonds and sauté until golden brown.
4. Add minced garlic and sauté for an additional minute.
5. Toss the blanched green beans in the skillet, coating them with the almond and garlic mixture.
6. Drizzle with lemon juice, season with salt and pepper, and serve.

**Nutritional Information:**

- Calories: 120
- Protein: 4g
- Fat: 9g
- Carbohydrates: 10g
- Fiber: 5g

# Cucumber and Avocado Salad

**Prep Time:** 10 minutes
**Cook Time:** 0 minutes
**Serving Size:** 4

**Ingredients:**

- 2 cucumbers, sliced

- 2 avocados, diced

- 1/4 cup red onion, thinly sliced

- 1/4 cup fresh cilantro, chopped

- Juice of 2 limes

- Salt and pepper to taste

**Instructions:**

1. In a large bowl, combine sliced cucumbers, diced avocados, red onion, and chopped cilantro.

2. Drizzle with lime juice and toss gently.

3. Season with salt and pepper before serving.

**Nutritional Information:**

- Calories: 160

- Protein: 3g

- Fat: 14g

- Carbohydrates: 10g

- Fiber: 7g

**Prep Time:** 15 minutes
**Cook Time:** 30 minutes
**Serving Size:** 4

**Ingredients:**

- 3 sweet potatoes, peeled and diced
- 2 tablespoons olive oil
- 1 tablespoon fresh rosemary, chopped
- 1 tablespoon fresh thyme, chopped
- 1 tablespoon fresh parsley, chopped
- Salt and pepper to taste

**Instructions:**

1. Preheat the oven to 425°F (220°C).
2. In a bowl, toss sweet potatoes with olive oil, chopped rosemary, thyme, parsley, salt, and pepper.
3. Spread on a baking sheet and roast for 30 minutes or until tender.
4. Serve hot.

**Nutritional Information:**

- Calories: 160
- Protein: 2g
- Fat: 7g
- Carbohydrates: 25g
- Fiber: 4g

## Spinach and Mushroom Quiche

**Prep Time:** 20 minutes

**Cook Time:** 40 minutes

**Serving Size:** 6

**Ingredients:**

- 1 pie crust (whole wheat or alternative)

- 2 cups spinach, chopped

- 1 cup mushrooms, sliced

- 1/2 cup feta cheese, crumbled

- 4 eggs

- 1 cup almond milk

- 1 teaspoon olive oil

- Salt and pepper to taste

**Instructions:**

1. Preheat the oven to 375°F (190°C).

2. In a skillet, sauté chopped spinach and sliced mushrooms with olive oil until wilted.

3. In a bowl, whisk together eggs, almond milk, salt, and pepper.

4. Place the pie crust in a pie dish and layer with sautéed spinach and mushrooms. Sprinkle feta cheese on top.

5. Pour the egg mixture over the vegetables and cheese.

6. Bake for 40 minutes or until the quiche is set and golden brown.

**Nutritional Information:**

- Calories: 220

- Protein: 10g

- Fat: 15g

- Carbohydrates: 15g

- Fiber: 3g

**Prep Time:** 10 minutes

**Cook Time:** 25 minutes

**Serving Size:** 4

**Ingredients:**

- 1 head cauliflower, cut into florets

- 2 tablespoons white miso paste

- 1 tablespoon sesame oil

- 1 tablespoon soy sauce

- 1 tablespoon maple syrup

- 1 teaspoon ginger, grated

- 2 green onions, sliced

- Sesame seeds for garnish

**Instructions:**

1. Preheat the oven to 425°F (220°C).

2. In a bowl, whisk together miso paste, sesame oil, soy sauce, maple syrup, and grated ginger.

3. Toss cauliflower florets with the miso glaze.

4. Spread on a baking sheet and roast for 25 minutes or until golden and caramelized.

5. Garnish with sliced green onions and sesame seeds before serving.

**Nutritional Information:**

- Calories: 120

- Protein: 5g

- Fat: 6g

- Carbohydrates: 15g

- Fiber: 5g

Miso-Glazed Roasted Cauliflower

# Brussels Sprouts and Apple Slaw

**Prep Time:** 15 minutes

**Cook Time:** 0 minutes

**Serving Size:** 4

**Ingredients:**

- 1 lb Brussels sprouts, thinly sliced

- 2 apples, julienned

- 1/2 cup dried cranberries

- 1/4 cup almonds, sliced

- 1/4 cup Greek yogurt

- 2 tablespoons apple cider vinegar

- 1 tablespoon honey

- Salt and pepper to taste

**Instructions:**

1. In a large bowl, combine sliced Brussels sprouts, julienned apples, dried cranberries, and sliced almonds.

2. In a small bowl, whisk together Greek yogurt, apple cider vinegar, honey, salt, and pepper.

3. Pour the dressing over the slaw and toss until well coated.

4. Chill before serving.

**Nutritional Information:**

- Calories: 180

- Protein: 5g

- Fat: 8g

- Carbohydrates: 25g

- Fiber: 7g

Brussels Sprouts and Apple Slaw

**Prep Time:** 15 minutes

**Cook Time:** 40 minutes

**Serving Size:** 4

**Ingredients:**

- 1 medium spaghetti squash

- 1 cup cherry tomatoes, halved

- 1/4 cup pine nuts, toasted

- 1/2 cup fresh basil, chopped

- 1/3 cup Pecorino Romano cheese, grated

- 2 tablespoons olive oil

- Salt and pepper to taste

**Instructions:**

1. Preheat the oven to 400°F (200°C).

2. Cut the spaghetti squash in half lengthwise and scoop out the seeds.

3. Drizzle with olive oil, season with salt and pepper, and place cut-side down on a baking sheet.

4. Roast for 40 minutes or until the squash is tender.

5. Scrape the spaghetti squash into strands using a fork and toss with cherry tomatoes, pine nuts, chopped basil, and Pecorino Romano cheese.

**Nutritional Information:**

- Calories: 220

- Protein: 6g

- Fat: 14g

- Carbohydrates: 20g

- Fiber: 5g

Spaghetti Squash with Pesto and Cherry Tomatoes

**Prep Time:** 10 minutes
**Cook Time:** 10 minutes
**Serving Size:** 4

**Ingredients:**

- 1 head cauliflower, grated

- 2 tablespoons olive oil

- 1/4 cup fresh cilantro, chopped

- Zest and juice of 1 lime

- 1/2 teaspoon cumin

- Salt and pepper to taste

**Instructions:**

1. In a large skillet, heat olive oil over medium heat.

2. Add grated cauliflower and sauté for 5-7 minutes until tender.

3. Stir in chopped cilantro, lime zest, lime juice, cumin, salt, and pepper.

4. Cook for an additional 2-3 minutes before serving.

**Nutritional Information:**

- Calories: 90

- Protein: 3g

- Fat: 7g

- Carbohydrates: 8g

- Fiber: 4g

Cilantro Lime Cauliflower Rice

# Chapter 5: Fish and seafood

## Lemon Herb Baked Salmon

**Prep Time:** 10 minutes
**Cook Time:** 15 minutes
**Serving Size:** 4

**Ingredients:**

- 4 salmon fillets

- 2 tablespoons olive oil

- Zest and juice of 1 lemon

- 2 cloves garlic, minced

- 1 tablespoon fresh dill, chopped

- Salt and pepper to taste

**Instructions:**

1. Preheat the oven to 400°F (200°C).

2. Place salmon fillets on a baking sheet.

3. In a bowl, mix olive oil, lemon zest, lemon juice, minced garlic, fresh dill, salt, and pepper.

4. Brush the mixture over the salmon.

5. Bake for 15 minutes or until the salmon is cooked through.

**Nutritional Information:**

- Calories: 250

- Protein: 25g

- Fat: 15g

- Carbohydrates: 2g

- Fiber: 0g

**Prep Time:** 15 minutes

**Cook Time:** 5 minutes

**Serving Size:** 4

**Ingredients:**

- 1 lb large shrimp, peeled and deveined

- 3 tablespoons unsalted butter, melted

- 3 cloves garlic, minced

- 1 tablespoon fresh parsley, chopped

- Lemon wedges for serving

- Wooden skewers, soaked in water

**Instructions:**

1. Preheat the grill or grill pan.

2. In a bowl, combine melted butter, minced garlic, and chopped parsley.

3. Thread shrimp onto skewers.

4. Grill shrimp skewers for 2-3 minutes on each side, basting with the garlic butter mixture.

5. Serve with lemon wedges.

**Nutritional Information:**

- Calories: 180

- Protein: 20g

- Fat: 10g

- Carbohydrates: 1g

- Fiber: 0g

**Prep Time:** 15 minutes
**Cook Time:** 10 minutes
**Serving Size:** 6 tacos

**Ingredients:**

- 6 tilapia fillets

- 2 tablespoons blackened seasoning

- 1 tablespoon olive oil

- 6 whole-grain or corn tortillas

- Cabbage slaw (shredded cabbage, Greek yogurt, lime juice)

- Fresh cilantro for garnish

**Instructions:**

1. Rub tilapia fillets with blackened seasoning.

2. Heat olive oil in a skillet over medium-high heat.

3. Cook tilapia for 3-4 minutes per side or until fully cooked.

4. Warm tortillas and assemble tacos with tilapia, cabbage slaw, and fresh cilantro.

**Nutritional Information:**

- Calories: 200

- Protein: 20g

- Fat: 8g

- Carbohydrates: 15g

- Fiber: 3g

# Grilled Swordfish with Mango Salsa

**Prep Time:** 20 minutes

**Cook Time:** 10 minutes

**Serving Size:** 4

**Ingredients:**

- 4 swordfish steaks

- 2 tablespoons olive oil

- 1 teaspoon cumin

- 1 teaspoon paprika

- Salt and pepper to taste

- Mango Salsa: mango, red onion, jalapeño, cilantro, lime juice

**Instructions:**

1. Preheat the grill.

2. Rub swordfish steaks with olive oil, cumin, paprika, salt, and pepper.

3. Grill swordfish for 4-5 minutes per side or until grill marks appear.

4. Prepare mango salsa by combining diced mango, red onion, jalapeño, cilantro, and lime juice.

5. Serve grilled swordfish topped with mango salsa.

**Nutritional Information:**

- Calories: 280

- Protein: 30g

- Fat: 12g

- Carbohydrates: 15g

- Fiber: 2g

Grilled Swordfish with Mango Salsa

**Prep Time:** 15 minutes
**Cook Time:** 5 minutes
**Serving Size:** 4

**Ingredients:**

- 1 lb shrimp, peeled and deveined

- 2 tablespoons olive oil

- Zest and juice of 2 limes

- 2 tablespoons fresh cilantro, chopped

- 1 teaspoon honey

- Mixed salad greens

**Instructions:**

1. In a bowl, toss shrimp with olive oil, lime zest, lime juice, chopped cilantro, and honey.

2. Heat a skillet over medium-high heat and cook shrimp for 2-3 minutes per side.

3. Serve shrimp over a bed of mixed salad greens.

**Nutritional Information:**

- Calories: 180

- Protein: 20g

- Fat: 8g

- Carbohydrates: 5g

- Fiber: 2g

# Coconut-Crusted Mahi-Mahi

**Prep Time:** 20 minutes

**Cook Time:** 15 minutes

**Serving Size:** 4

**Ingredients:**

- 4 mahi-mahi fillets

- 1/2 cup unsweetened shredded coconut

- 1/4 cup almond flour

- 1 teaspoon paprika

- 1/2 teaspoon garlic powder

- 2 eggs, beaten

- 2 tablespoons coconut oil

- Lime wedges for serving

**Instructions:**

1. Preheat the oven to 400°F (200°C).

2. In a shallow dish, mix shredded coconut, almond flour, paprika, and garlic powder.

3. Dip mahi-mahi fillets in beaten eggs, then coat with the coconut mixture.

4. Heat coconut oil in an oven-safe skillet over medium-high heat.

5. Sear mahi-mahi for 2 minutes per side, then transfer the skillet to the oven and bake for an additional 10 minutes.

6. Serve with lime wedges.

**Nutritional Information:**

- Calories: 320

- Protein: 25g

- Fat: 20g

- Carbohydrates: 10g

- Fiber: 5g

**Prep Time:** 15 minutes

**Cook Time:** 20 minutes

**Serving Size:** 4

**Ingredients:**

- 1 lb shrimp, peeled and deveined

- 2 tablespoons Cajun seasoning

- 1 cup quinoa, cooked

- 1 cup cherry tomatoes, halved

- 1 avocado, sliced

- 1/4 cup Greek yogurt

- Fresh cilantro for garnish

**Instructions:**

1. Toss shrimp with Cajun seasoning in a bowl.

2. Cook shrimp in a skillet over medium-high heat for 2-3 minutes per side.

3. Assemble bowls with cooked quinoa, Cajun shrimp, cherry tomatoes, avocado slices, and a dollop of Greek yogurt.

4. Garnish with fresh cilantro before serving.

**Nutritional Information:**

- Calories: 350

- Protein: 30g

- Fat: 15g

- Carbohydrates: 25g

- Fiber: 5g

**Prep Time:** 15 minutes

**Cook Time:** 15 minutes

**Serving Size:** 4

**Ingredients:**

- 4 cod fillets

- 1/2 cup whole wheat breadcrumbs

- 2 tablespoons fresh parsley, chopped

- 1 tablespoon fresh dill, chopped

- 1 teaspoon lemon zest

- Salt and pepper to taste

- Lemon Dill Sauce: Greek yogurt, lemon juice, dill, garlic

**Instructions:**

1. Preheat the oven to 400°F (200°C).

2. In a bowl, combine breadcrumbs, chopped parsley, chopped dill, lemon zest, salt, and pepper.

3. Press the breadcrumb mixture onto each cod fillet.

4. Bake cod in the oven for 15 minutes or until golden and flaky.

5. Prepare Lemon Dill Sauce by mixing Greek yogurt, lemon juice, chopped dill, and minced garlic.

6. Serve cod fillets with a drizzle of Lemon Dill Sauce.

**Nutritional Information:**

- Calories: 220

- Protein: 25g

- Fat: 5g

- Carbohydrates: 15g

- Fiber: 3g

**Prep Time:** 10 minutes
**Cook Time:** 15 minutes
**Serving Size:** 4

**Ingredients:**

- 4 salmon fillets

- 1/4 cup soy sauce

- 2 tablespoons sesame oil

- 1 tablespoon honey

- 1 tablespoon rice vinegar

- 1 teaspoon fresh ginger, grated

- Sesame seeds for garnish

- Green onions, sliced, for garnish

**Instructions:**

1. In a bowl, whisk together soy sauce, sesame oil, honey, rice vinegar, and grated ginger.

2. Place salmon fillets in a dish and pour the marinade over them. Let it marinate for 10 minutes.

3. Preheat the grill or grill pan.

4. Grill salmon for 3-4 minutes per side or until cooked through.

5. Garnish with sesame seeds and sliced green onions before serving.

**Nutritional Information:**

- Calories: 280

- Protein: 30g

- Fat: 15g

- Carbohydrates: 10g

- Fiber: 1g

**Prep Time:** 20 minutes

**Cook Time:** 0 minutes

**Serving Size:** 4

**Ingredients:**

- 1 lb white fish (cod, halibut), diced

- 2 mangoes, diced

- 1 red onion, finely chopped

- 1 jalapeño, seeded and minced

- 1/4 cup fresh cilantro, chopped

- Juice of 3 limes

- Salt and pepper to taste

- Tortilla chips for serving

**Instructions:**

1. In a bowl, combine diced white fish, diced mangoes, chopped red onion, minced jalapeño, chopped cilantro, lime juice, salt, and pepper.

2. Mix well and refrigerate for at least 15 minutes to let flavors meld.

3. Serve chilled with tortilla chips.

**Nutritional Information:**

- Calories: 220

- Protein: 25g

- Fat: 5g

- Carbohydrates: 20g

- Fiber: 3g

**Prep Time:** 15 minutes

**Cook Time:** 10 minutes

**Serving Size:** 4

**Ingredients:**

- 4 halibut fillets

- 3 tablespoons olive oil

- Zest and juice of 2 limes

- 2 cloves garlic, minced

- 1/4 cup fresh cilantro, chopped

- Salt and pepper to taste

**Instructions:**

1. Preheat the grill.

2. In a bowl, mix olive oil, lime zest, lime juice, minced garlic, chopped cilantro, salt, and pepper.

3. Brush the mixture over halibut fillets.

4. Grill for 4-5 minutes on each side or until the halibut is cooked through.

5. Serve with extra cilantro lime sauce.

**Nutritional Information:**

- Calories: 250

- Protein: 30g

- Fat: 14g

- Carbohydrates: 2g

- Fiber: 0g

Shrimp and Avocado Salad

**Prep Time:** 15 minutes

**Cook Time:** 5 minutes

**Serving Size:** 4

**Ingredients:**

- 1 lb shrimp, peeled and deveined

- 2 avocados, diced

- 1 cup cherry tomatoes, halved

- 1/4 cup red onion, finely chopped

- 1/4 cup fresh cilantro, chopped

- 2 tablespoons olive oil

- Zest and juice of 1 lime

- Salt and pepper to taste

**Instructions:**

1. Cook shrimp in a skillet over medium-high heat for 2-3 minutes per side.

2. In a large bowl, combine cooked shrimp, diced avocados, cherry tomatoes, red onion, and chopped cilantro.

3. In a small bowl, whisk together olive oil, lime zest, lime juice, salt, and pepper.

4. Drizzle the dressing over the shrimp and avocado mixture.

5. Toss gently and serve immediately.

**Nutritional Information:**

- Calories: 280

- Protein: 25g

- Fat: 18g

- Carbohydrates: 12g

- Fiber: 6g

# Coconut Lime Grilled Snapper

**Prep Time:** 20 minutes
**Cook Time:** 10 minutes
**Serving Size:** 4

**Ingredients:**

- 4 snapper fillets

- 1/2 cup coconut milk

- Zest and juice of 2 limes

- 2 tablespoons fresh cilantro, chopped

- 1 tablespoon soy sauce

- 1 tablespoon honey

- Salt and pepper to taste

**Instructions:**

1. In a bowl, whisk together coconut milk, lime zest, lime juice, chopped cilantro, soy sauce, honey, salt, and pepper.

2. Marinate snapper fillets in the mixture for 15 minutes.

3. Preheat the grill.

4. Grill snapper for 4-5 minutes on each side or until the fish is opaque.

5. Serve with extra marinade.

**Nutritional Information:**

- Calories: 220

- Protein: 25g

- Fat: 10g

- Carbohydrates: 8g

- Fiber: 1g

**Prep Time:** 15 minutes

**Cook Time:** 10 minutes

**Serving Size:** 6 tacos

**Ingredients:**

- 6 catfish fillets

- 2 tablespoons Cajun seasoning

- 1 tablespoon olive oil

- 6 whole-grain or corn tortillas

- Cabbage slaw (shredded cabbage, Greek yogurt, lime juice)

- Fresh cilantro for garnish

**Instructions:**

1. Rub catfish fillets with Cajun seasoning.

2. Heat olive oil in a skillet over medium-high heat.

3. Cook catfish for 3-4 minutes per side or until fully cooked.

4. Warm tortillas and assemble tacos with catfish, cabbage slaw, and fresh cilantro.

**Nutritional Information:**

- Calories: 240

- Protein: 20g

- Fat: 10g

- Carbohydrates: 15g

- Fiber: 3g

**Prep Time:** 25 minutes

**Cook Time:** 15 minutes

**Serving Size:** 4

**Ingredients:**

- 4 trout fillets

- 1/2 cup pecans, finely chopped

- 2 tablespoons fresh parsley, chopped

- 1 tablespoon Dijon mustard

- 1 tablespoon olive oil

- Zest and juice of 1 lemon

- Salt and pepper to taste

**Instructions:**

1. Preheat the grill.

2. In a bowl, combine chopped pecans, chopped parsley, Dijon mustard, olive oil, lemon zest, lemon juice, salt, and pepper.

3. Press the pecan mixture onto each trout fillet.

4. Grill trout for 4-5 minutes on each side or until the fish flakes easily.

5. Serve with a squeeze of lemon.

**Nutritional Information:**

- Calories: 280

- Protein: 30g

- Fat: 18g

- Carbohydrates: 4g

- Fiber: 2g

Herb-Grilled Trout with Pecan Crust

# Chapter 6: Beef, pork, and lamb



## Grilled Rosemary Garlic Lamb Chops

**Prep Time:** 15 minutes
**Cook Time:** 10 minutes
**Serving Size:** 4

**Ingredients:**

- 8 lamb chops

- 2 tablespoons olive oil

- 3 cloves garlic, minced

- 2 tablespoons fresh rosemary, chopped

- Salt and pepper to taste

**Instructions:**

1. Preheat the grill.

2. In a bowl, mix olive oil, minced garlic, chopped rosemary, salt, and pepper.

3. Brush the mixture over lamb chops.

4. Grill lamb chops for 4-5 minutes per side or until desired doneness.

5. Serve immediately.

**Nutritional Information:**

- Calories: 300

- Protein: 25g

- Fat: 20g

- Carbohydrates: 0g

- Fiber: 0g

**Prep Time:** 20 minutes
**Cook Time:** 6 hours (slow cooker)
**Serving Size:** 6 tacos

**Ingredients:**

- 2 lbs pork shoulder, trimmed

- 1 can (7 oz) chipotle peppers in adobo sauce

- 1 onion, sliced

- 3 cloves garlic, minced

- 1 tablespoon cumin

- 1 tablespoon smoked paprika

- 6 whole-grain or corn tortillas

- Cilantro and lime wedges for garnish

**Instructions:**

1. Place pork shoulder in a slow cooker.

2. Blend chipotle peppers with adobo sauce, sliced onion, minced garlic, cumin, and smoked paprika.

3. Pour the chipotle mixture over the pork.

4. Cook on low for 6 hours or until pork is tender and easy to shred.

5. Serve pulled pork in tortillas with cilantro and lime wedges.

**Nutritional Information:**

- Calories: 350

- Protein: 30g

- Fat: 20g

- Carbohydrates: 15g

- Fiber: 3g

Spicy Chipotle Pulled Pork Tacos

# Mint and Balsamic Glazed Lamb Kebabs

**Prep Time:** 20 minutes
**Cook Time:** 15 minutes
**Serving Size:** 4

**Ingredients:**

- 1 lb lamb cubes

- 2 tablespoons balsamic vinegar

- 2 tablespoons olive oil

- 2 tablespoons fresh mint, chopped

- 1 tablespoon honey

- Salt and pepper to taste

**Instructions:**

1. Preheat the grill.

2. In a bowl, mix balsamic vinegar, olive oil, chopped mint, honey, salt, and pepper.

3. Thread lamb cubes onto skewers.

4. Grill lamb kebabs for 6-8 minutes, turning occasionally and basting with the balsamic mixture.

5. Serve with extra glaze on the side.

**Nutritional Information:**

- Calories: 280

- Protein: 25g

- Fat: 18g

- Carbohydrates: 5g

- Fiber: 0g

**Prep Time:** 10 minutes

**Cook Time:** 25 minutes

**Serving Size:** 4

**Ingredients:**

- 2 pork tenderloins

- 1/4 cup Dijon mustard

- 2 tablespoons honey

- 1 tablespoon olive oil

- 2 cloves garlic, minced

- Salt and pepper to taste

**Instructions:**

1. Preheat the oven to 400°F (200°C).

2. In a bowl, whisk together Dijon mustard, honey, olive oil, minced garlic, salt, and pepper.

3. Coat pork tenderloins with the honey mustard mixture.

4. Roast in the oven for 25 minutes or until the internal temperature reaches 145°F (63°C).

5. Let it rest for 5 minutes before slicing.

**Nutritional Information:**

- Calories: 320

- Protein: 30g

- Fat: 12g

- Carbohydrates: 15g

- Fiber: 1g

**Prep Time:** 15 minutes
**Cook Time:** 10 minutes
**Serving Size:** 4

**Ingredients:**

- 1 lb beef tenderloin medallions

- 3 cloves garlic, minced

- 2 tablespoons fresh thyme, chopped

- 2 tablespoons olive oil

- Salt and pepper to taste

**Instructions:**

1. In a bowl, mix minced garlic, chopped thyme, olive oil, salt, and pepper.

2. Coat beef medallions with the garlic herb mixture.

3. Heat a skillet over medium-high heat.

4. Cook beef medallions for 3-4 minutes per side or until desired doneness.

5. Let it rest for a few minutes before serving.

**Nutritional Information:**

- Calories: 280

- Protein: 30g

- Fat: 16g

- Carbohydrates: 0g

- Fiber: 0g

# Lemon Rosemary Grilled Lamb Burgers

**Prep Time:** 20 minutes

**Cook Time:** 12 minutes

**Serving Size:** 4

**Ingredients:**

- 1 lb ground lamb

- 2 tablespoons fresh rosemary, chopped

- Zest and juice of 1 lemon

- 1/4 cup feta cheese, crumbled

- 4 whole-grain burger buns

- Lettuce, tomato, and red onion for garnish

**Instructions:**

1. Preheat the grill.

2. In a bowl, combine ground lamb, chopped rosemary, lemon zest, lemon juice, and crumbled feta.

3. Form the mixture into patties.

4. Grill lamb burgers for 5-6 minutes per side or until fully cooked.

5. Serve on whole-grain buns with lettuce, tomato, and red onion.

**Nutritional Information:**

- Calories: 350

- Protein: 20g

- Fat: 25g

- Carbohydrates: 20g

- Fiber: 3g

**Prep Time:** 15 minutes

**Cook Time:** 12 minutes

**Serving Size:** 4

**Ingredients:**

- 4 pork chops

- 2 tablespoons chili powder

- Zest and juice of 2 limes

- 1 tablespoon olive oil

- 1 teaspoon cayenne pepper (optional)

- Salt and pepper to taste

**Instructions:**

1. Preheat the grill.

2. In a bowl, mix chili powder, lime zest, lime juice, olive oil, cayenne pepper (if using), salt, and pepper.

3. Brush the mixture over pork chops.

4. Grill pork chops for 5-6 minutes per side or until the internal temperature reaches 145°F (63°C).

5. Let them rest for a few minutes before serving.

**Nutritional Information:**

- Calories: 300

- Protein: 25g

- Fat: 18g

- Carbohydrates: 5g

- Fiber: 1g

**Prep Time:** 30 minutes
**Cook Time:** 30 minutes
**Serving Size:** 6

**Ingredients:**

- 1 lb ground lamb

- 1 cup quinoa, cooked

- 1 can (14 oz) diced tomatoes, drained

- 1/2 cup Kalamata olives, chopped

- 1/4 cup feta cheese, crumbled

- 6 bell peppers, halved and seeded

- 2 tablespoons olive oil

- Fresh parsley for garnish

**Instructions:**

1. Preheat the oven to 375°F (190°C).

2. In a skillet, brown ground lamb over medium-high heat.

3. In a large bowl, combine cooked quinoa, diced tomatoes, chopped olives, and crumbled feta.

4. Stir in the browned lamb.

5. Brush bell pepper halves with olive oil and stuff them with the lamb and quinoa mixture.

6. Bake for 25-30 minutes or until peppers are tender.

7. Garnish with fresh parsley before serving.

**Nutritional Information:**

- Calories: 320

- Protein: 25g

- Fat: 18g

- Carbohydrates: 20g

- Fiber: 5g

## Balsamic Glazed Beef Skewers

**Prep Time:** 25 minutes
**Cook Time:** 10 minutes
**Serving Size:** 4

**Ingredients:**

- 1 lb beef sirloin, cubed

- 1/4 cup balsamic vinegar

- 2 tablespoons olive oil

- 1 tablespoon Dijon mustard

- 1 tablespoon honey

- 2 cloves garlic, minced

- Salt and pepper to taste

**Instructions:**

1. In a bowl, whisk together balsamic vinegar, olive oil, Dijon mustard, honey, minced garlic, salt, and pepper.

2. Marinate beef cubes in the balsamic mixture for at least 20 minutes.

3. Thread marinated beef onto skewers.

4. Grill beef skewers for 3-4 minutes per side or until cooked to your liking.

5. Serve with extra balsamic glaze.

**Nutritional Information:**

- Calories: 280

- Protein: 30g

- Fat: 15g

- Carbohydrates: 8g

- Fiber: 1g

**Prep Time:** 15 minutes

**Cook Time:** 1 hour

**Serving Size:** 6

**Ingredients:**

- 2 lbs pork loin

- 1 cup apple cider

- 1 onion, sliced

- 2 apples, sliced

- 2 tablespoons whole-grain mustard

- 1 tablespoon thyme leaves

- Salt and pepper to taste

**Instructions:**

1. Preheat the oven to 350°F (175°C).

2. Season pork loin with salt and pepper.

3. In a Dutch oven, brown pork loin on all sides over medium-high heat.

4. Add sliced onion and apples around the pork.

5. Mix apple cider, whole-grain mustard, and thyme leaves. Pour over the pork.

6. Cover and bake for 1 hour or until the internal temperature reaches 145°F (63°C).

7. Let it rest before slicing.

**Nutritional Information:**

- Calories: 320

- Protein: 30g

- Fat: 15g

- Carbohydrates: 15g

- Fiber: 2g

**Prep Time:** 20 minutes

**Cook Time:** 1 hour

**Serving Size:** 6

**Ingredients:**

- 1.5 lbs beef stew meat, cubed

- 1 onion, diced

- 2 bell peppers, diced

- 3 cloves garlic, minced

- 2 teaspoons cumin

- 1 teaspoon smoked paprika

- 1 can (15 oz) black beans, drained and rinsed

- 1 can (14 oz) diced tomatoes

- 4 cups beef broth

- Salt and pepper to taste

- Fresh cilantro for garnish

**Instructions:**

1. In a Dutch oven, brown beef stew meat over medium-high heat.

2. Add diced onion, bell peppers, and minced garlic. Sauté until vegetables are softened.

3. Stir in cumin, smoked paprika, black beans, diced tomatoes, and beef broth.

4. Season with salt and pepper.

5. Simmer for 1 hour or until beef is tender.

6. Garnish with fresh cilantro before serving.

**Nutritional Information:**

- Calories: 350

- Protein: 30g

- Fat: 12g

- Carbohydrates: 25g

- Fiber: 8g

## Mango Habanero Glazed Pork Ribs

**Prep Time:** 15 minutes
**Cook Time:** 2 hours (oven or grill)
**Serving Size:** 4

**Ingredients:**

- 2 racks of pork ribs

- 1 cup mango puree

- 2 tablespoons apple cider vinegar

- 1 habanero pepper, minced

- 1/4 cup brown sugar

- 2 teaspoons smoked paprika

- Salt and pepper to taste

**Instructions:**

1. Preheat the oven to 300°F (150°C) or prepare a grill for indirect heat.

2. In a bowl, mix mango puree, apple cider vinegar, minced habanero pepper, brown sugar, smoked paprika, salt, and pepper.

3. Rub the mixture over both sides of the pork ribs.

4. Roast in the oven or grill over indirect heat for 2 hours or until the ribs are tender.

5. Baste with additional glaze during the last 30 minutes of cooking.

6. Let them rest before slicing.

**Nutritional Information:**

- Calories: 420

- Protein: 25g

- Fat: 30g

- Carbohydrates: 20g

- Fiber: 2g

## Herbed Lamb Meatballs with Tzatziki Sauce

**Prep Time:** 25 minutes
**Cook Time:** 20 minutes
**Serving Size:** 5

**Ingredients:**

- 1 lb ground lamb

- 1/2 cup breadcrumbs

- 1/4 cup fresh mint, chopped

- 1/4 cup fresh parsley, chopped

- 1 teaspoon cumin

- 1 teaspoon coriander

- 1/2 teaspoon cinnamon

- Salt and pepper to taste

- Tzatziki Sauce: Greek yogurt, cucumber, garlic, dill

**Instructions:**

1. Preheat the oven to 375°F (190°C).

2. In a bowl, combine ground lamb, breadcrumbs, chopped mint, chopped parsley, cumin, coriander, cinnamon, salt, and pepper.

3. Shape the mixture into meatballs and place on a baking sheet.

4. Bake for 20 minutes or until the meatballs are cooked through.

5. Prepare Tzatziki Sauce by combining Greek yogurt, diced cucumber, minced garlic, and chopped dill.

6. Serve meatballs with Tzatziki Sauce.

**Nutritional Information:**

- Calories: 320

- Protein: 20g

- Fat: 25g

- Carbohydrates: 10g

- Fiber: 2g

## Sage and Apple Stuffed Pork Tenderloin

**Prep Time:** 30 minutes
**Cook Time:** 25 minutes
**Serving Size:** 4

**Ingredients:**

- 2 pork tenderloins

- 1 cup apple, finely diced

- 1/2 cup breadcrumbs

- 2 tablespoons fresh sage, chopped

- 2 tablespoons olive oil

- 1 tablespoon Dijon mustard

- Salt and pepper to taste

**Instructions:**

1. Preheat the oven to 400°F (200°C).

2. In a bowl, mix diced apple, breadcrumbs, chopped sage, olive oil, Dijon mustard, salt, and pepper.

3. Butterfly each pork tenderloin and fill with the apple stuffing.

4. Secure with kitchen twine.

5. Roast in the oven for 25 minutes or until the internal temperature reaches 145°F (63°C).

6. Let it rest before slicing.

**Nutritional Information:**

- Calories: 280

- Protein: 30g

- Fat: 12g

- Carbohydrates: 15g

- Fiber: 2g

## Moroccan Spiced Beef Skewers

**Prep Time:** 20 minutes
**Cook Time:** 10 minutes
**Serving Size:** 4

**Ingredients:**

- 1.5 lbs beef sirloin, cubed

- 2 tablespoons Moroccan spice blend

- 1/4 cup plain Greek yogurt

- 2 tablespoons olive oil

- 1 tablespoon lemon juice

- Salt and pepper to taste

**Instructions:**

1. In a bowl, mix Moroccan spice blend, Greek yogurt, olive oil, lemon juice, salt, and pepper.

2. Marinate beef cubes in the mixture for at least 15 minutes.

3. Thread marinated beef onto skewers.

4. Grill beef skewers for 3-4 minutes per side or until cooked to your liking.

5. Serve with a side of Greek yogurt sauce.

**Nutritional Information:**

- Calories: 340

- Protein: 25g

- Fat: 18g

- Carbohydrates: 5g

- Fiber: 1g

# Chapter 7: Poultry and mains



**Prep Time:** 15 minutes
**Cook Time:** 1.5 hours
**Serving Size:** 4

**Ingredients:**

- 1 whole chicken (about 4 lbs)

- 2 lemons, sliced

- 3 cloves garlic, minced

- 2 tablespoons fresh rosemary, chopped

- 2 tablespoons olive oil

- Salt and pepper to taste

**Instructions:**

1. Preheat the oven to 375°F (190°C).

2. Rinse and pat dry the whole chicken.

3. In a bowl, mix minced garlic, chopped rosemary, olive oil, salt, and pepper.

4. Rub the mixture over the chicken, including under the skin.

5. Stuff the cavity with lemon slices.

6. Roast in the oven for 1.5 hours or until the internal temperature reaches 165°F (74°C).

7. Let it rest before carving.

**Nutritional Information:**

- Calories: 300

- Protein: 25g

- Fat: 20g

- Carbohydrates: 2g

- Fiber: 1g

**Prep Time:** 20 minutes

**Cook Time:** 40 minutes

**Serving Size:** 6

**Ingredients:**

- 2 lbs turkey breast

- 1 cup mango, diced

- 1 jalapeño, minced

- 2 tablespoons lime juice

- 1 tablespoon honey

- 1 teaspoon cumin

- Salt and pepper to taste

**Instructions:**

1. Preheat the grill.

2. In a bowl, combine diced mango, minced jalapeño, lime juice, honey, cumin, salt, and pepper.

3. Brush the mixture over the turkey breast.

4. Grill turkey breast for 20 minutes per side or until the internal temperature reaches 165°F (74°C).

5. Let it rest before slicing.

**Nutritional Information:**

- Calories: 280

- Protein: 30g

- Fat: 10g

- Carbohydrates: 10g

- Fiber: 1g

# Crispy Baked Pecan-Crusted Chicken Tenders

**Prep Time:** 15 minutes
**Cook Time:** 20 minutes
**Serving Size:** 4

**Ingredients:**

- 1 lb chicken tenders

- 1 cup pecans, finely chopped

- 1/2 cup whole wheat flour

- 2 eggs, beaten

- 1 teaspoon smoked paprika

- Salt and pepper to taste

**Instructions:**

1. Preheat the oven to 400°F (200°C).

2. In a shallow dish, mix chopped pecans, whole wheat flour, smoked paprika, salt, and pepper.

3. Dip each chicken tender in beaten eggs and coat with the pecan mixture.

4. Place on a baking sheet and bake for 20 minutes or until golden and crispy.

5. Serve with a dipping sauce of your choice.

**Nutritional Information:**

- Calories: 320

- Protein: 25g

- Fat: 20g

- Carbohydrates: 10g

- Fiber: 3g

**Prep Time:** 30 minutes
**Cook Time:** 15 minutes
**Serving Size:** 4

**Ingredients:**

- 1.5 lbs chicken thighs, boneless and skinless, cut into cubes

- 1/2 cup coconut milk

- 2 tablespoons curry powder

- 1 tablespoon soy sauce

- 1 tablespoon honey

- 1 teaspoon ginger, grated

- Wooden skewers, soaked in water

**Instructions:**

1. In a bowl, mix coconut milk, curry powder, soy sauce, honey, and grated ginger.

2. Marinate chicken cubes in the mixture for at least 20 minutes.

3. Thread marinated chicken onto soaked wooden skewers.

4. Grill chicken skewers for 5-7 minutes per side or until fully cooked.

5. Serve with extra coconut curry sauce.

**Nutritional Information:**

- Calories: 350

- Protein: 30g

- Fat: 18g

- Carbohydrates: 8g

- Fiber: 1g

**Prep Time:** 25 minutes

**Cook Time:** 30 minutes

**Serving Size:** 4

**Ingredients:**

- 4 chicken breasts, boneless and skinless

- 2 cups spinach, chopped

- 1/2 cup feta cheese, crumbled

- 1/4 cup sun-dried tomatoes, chopped

- 2 cloves garlic, minced

- 1 tablespoon olive oil

- Salt and pepper to taste

**Instructions:**

1. Preheat the oven to 375°F (190°C).

2. In a skillet, sauté chopped spinach, crumbled feta, chopped sun-dried tomatoes, and minced garlic in olive oil until spinach wilts.

3. Butterfly each chicken breast and fill with the spinach and feta mixture.

4. Secure with toothpicks if needed.

5. Bake in the oven for 30 minutes or until the internal temperature reaches 165°F (74°C).

6. Let it rest before serving.

**Nutritional Information:**

- Calories: 320

- Protein: 30g

- Fat: 15g

- Carbohydrates: 5g

- Fiber: 2g

**Prep Time:** 20 minutes

**Cook Time:** 12 minutes

**Serving Size:** 4

**Ingredients:**

- 1.5 lbs ground turkey

- 1/4 cup whole grain mustard

- 2 tablespoons honey

- 1 tablespoon olive oil

- 1 teaspoon garlic powder

- Salt and pepper to taste

- Whole grain burger buns

- Lettuce, tomato, and red onion for garnish

**Instructions:**

1. In a bowl, combine ground turkey, whole grain mustard, honey, olive oil, garlic powder, salt, and pepper.

2. Form the mixture into burger patties.

3. Grill turkey burgers for 5-6 minutes per side or until fully cooked.

4. Serve on whole grain buns with lettuce, tomato, and red onion.

**Nutritional Information:**

- Calories: 290

- Protein: 25g

- Fat: 15g

- Carbohydrates: 15g

- Fiber: 3g

**Prep Time:** 20 minutes

**Cook Time:** 15 minutes

**Serving Size:** 4

**Ingredients:**

- 1.5 lbs chicken breast, thinly sliced

- 2 cups broccoli florets

- 1 bell pepper, thinly sliced

- 1 zucchini, thinly sliced

- 1/4 cup balsamic vinegar

- 2 tablespoons soy sauce

- 1 tablespoon honey

- 1 tablespoon cornstarch

- 2 tablespoons olive oil

**Instructions:**

1. In a bowl, whisk together balsamic vinegar, soy sauce, honey, and cornstarch.

2. In a wok or large skillet, heat olive oil over medium-high heat.

3. Stir-fry sliced chicken until browned.

4. Add broccoli, bell pepper, and zucchini. Stir-fry until vegetables are tender-crisp.

5. Pour in the balsamic mixture and toss everything to combine.

6. Serve over brown rice or quinoa.

**Nutritional Information:**

- Calories: 320

- Protein: 30g

- Fat: 12g

- Carbohydrates: 20g

- Fiber: 5g

## Lime and Cilantro Grilled Chicken Thighs

**Prep Time:** 15 minutes
**Cook Time:** 20 minutes
**Serving Size:** 4

**Ingredients:**

- 2 lbs chicken thighs, bone-in and skin-on

- Zest and juice of 2 limes

- 1/4 cup fresh cilantro, chopped

- 2 tablespoons olive oil

- 1 teaspoon cumin

- Salt and pepper to taste

**Instructions:**

1. Preheat the grill.

2. In a bowl, mix lime zest, lime juice, chopped cilantro, olive oil, cumin, salt, and pepper.

3. Rub the mixture over the chicken thighs.

4. Grill chicken thighs for 10-12 minutes per side or until fully cooked.

5. Let them rest before serving.

**Nutritional Information:**

- Calories: 350

- Protein: 25g

- Fat: 22g

- Carbohydrates: 2g

- Fiber: 0g

# Cajun Spiced Turkey and Quinoa Stuffed Peppers

**Prep Time:** 30 minutes

**Cook Time:** 30 minutes

**Serving Size:** 6

**Ingredients:**

- 1.5 lbs ground turkey

- 1 cup quinoa, cooked

- 1 can (14 oz) diced tomatoes, drained

- 1 onion, diced

- 2 celery stalks, diced

- 2 teaspoons Cajun seasoning

- 6 bell peppers, halved and seeded

- 2 tablespoons olive oil

- Fresh parsley for garnish

**Instructions:**

1. Preheat the oven to 375°F (190°C).

2. In a skillet, brown ground turkey in olive oil over medium-high heat.

3. Add diced onion and celery. Sauté until vegetables are softened.

4. Stir in cooked quinoa, diced tomatoes, and Cajun seasoning.

5. Brush bell pepper halves with olive oil and stuff them with the turkey and quinoa mixture.

6. Bake for 25-30 minutes or until peppers are tender.

7. Garnish with fresh parsley before serving.

**Nutritional Information:**

- Calories: 320

- Protein: 30g

- Fat: 15g

- Carbohydrates: 20g

- Fiber: 5g

## Teriyaki Glazed Chicken Drumsticks

**Prep Time:** 15 minutes
**Cook Time:** 30 minutes
**Serving Size:** 6

**Ingredients:**

- 2 lbs chicken drumsticks

- 1/2 cup low-sodium soy sauce

- 1/4 cup honey

- 2 tablespoons rice vinegar

- 1 teaspoon ginger, grated

- 2 cloves garlic, minced

- Sesame seeds and green onions for garnish

**Instructions:**

1. Preheat the oven to 400°F (200°C).

2. In a bowl, whisk together soy sauce, honey, rice vinegar, grated ginger, and minced garlic.

3. Place chicken drumsticks in a baking dish and pour the teriyaki mixture over them.

4. Bake for 30 minutes or until chicken is cooked through.

5. Garnish with sesame seeds and chopped green onions before serving.

**Nutritional Information:**

- Calories: 280

- Protein: 25g

- Fat: 12g

- Carbohydrates: 15g

- Fiber: 1g

# Almond-Crusted Turkey Cutlets

**Prep Time:** 15 minutes
**Cook Time:** 12 minutes
**Serving Size:** 4

**Ingredients:**

- 1.5 lbs turkey cutlets

- 1 cup almonds, finely ground

- 1/2 cup whole wheat flour

- 2 eggs, beaten

- 1 teaspoon smoked paprika

- Salt and pepper to taste

**Instructions:**

1. In a shallow dish, mix finely ground almonds, whole wheat flour, smoked paprika, salt, and pepper.

2. Dip each turkey cutlet in beaten eggs and coat with the almond mixture.

3. Heat a skillet over medium-high heat.

4. Cook turkey cutlets for 5-6 minutes per side or until golden and cooked through.

5. Serve with a squeeze of lemon.

**Nutritional Information:**

- Calories: 320

- Protein: 30g

- Fat: 18g

- Carbohydrates: 10g

- Fiber: 3g

**Prep Time:** 15 minutes

**Cook Time:** 20 minutes

**Serving Size:** 4

**Ingredients:**

- 4 duck breasts, skin-on

- 1 cup pomegranate juice

- 1/4 cup honey

- 2 tablespoons balsamic vinegar

- 1 teaspoon Dijon mustard

- Salt and pepper to taste

**Instructions:**

1. Preheat the oven to 400°F (200°C).

2. Score the skin of the duck breasts in a crosshatch pattern.

3. Season duck breasts with salt and pepper.

4. In a saucepan, mix pomegranate juice, honey, balsamic vinegar, and Dijon mustard. Simmer until it thickens.

5. Sear duck breasts, skin side down, in an oven-safe skillet for 3-4 minutes.

6. Flip and brush with the pomegranate glaze.

7. Transfer the skillet to the oven and roast for 15-20 minutes or until the internal temperature reaches 145°F (63°C).

8. Let it rest before slicing.

**Nutritional Information:**

- Calories: 380

- Protein: 25g

- Fat: 22g

- Carbohydrates: 20g

- Fiber: 1g

Mediterranean Grilled Chicken Salad

**Prep Time:** 25 minutes
**Cook Time:** 15 minutes
**Serving Size:** 4

**Ingredients:**

- 1.5 lbs chicken breasts, grilled and sliced

- 6 cups mixed greens

- 1 cup cherry tomatoes, halved

- 1 cucumber, sliced

- 1/2 cup Kalamata olives, sliced

- 1/4 cup feta cheese, crumbled

- 2 tablespoons olive oil

- 1 tablespoon red wine vinegar

- 1 teaspoon dried oregano

- Salt and pepper to taste

**Instructions:**

1. In a large bowl, toss together mixed greens, cherry tomatoes, cucumber, Kalamata olives, and feta cheese.

2. Top the salad with grilled and sliced chicken breasts.

3. In a small bowl, whisk together olive oil, red wine vinegar, dried oregano, salt, and pepper.

4. Drizzle the dressing over the salad before serving.

**Nutritional Information:**

- Calories: 320

- Protein: 30g

- Fat: 18g

- Carbohydrates: 15g

- Fiber: 5g

## Teriyaki Glazed Salmon with Quinoa

**Prep Time:** 20 minutes
**Cook Time:** 15 minutes
**Serving Size:** 4

**Ingredients:**

- 1.5 lbs salmon fillets

- 1/2 cup teriyaki sauce

- 1 cup quinoa, cooked

- 1 cup broccoli florets, steamed

- 1 carrot, julienned

- 2 green onions, sliced

- Sesame seeds for garnish

**Instructions:**

1. Preheat the oven to 400°F (200°C).

2. Place salmon fillets on a baking sheet and brush with teriyaki sauce.

3. Bake for 15 minutes or until salmon is cooked through.

4. In a bowl, assemble quinoa, steamed broccoli, and julienned carrot.

5. Top with teriyaki-glazed salmon.

6. Garnish with sliced green onions and sesame seeds.

**Nutritional Information:**

- Calories: 350

- Protein: 25g

- Fat: 18g

- Carbohydrates: 25g

- Fiber: 4g

**Prep Time:** 15 minutes
**Cook Time:** 20 minutes
**Serving Size:** 4

**Ingredients:**

- 1.5 lbs large shrimp, peeled and deveined

- 1 tablespoon Cajun seasoning

- 2 tablespoons olive oil

- 2 cups brown rice, cooked

- 1 bell pepper, diced

- 1 red onion, diced

- 1 cup corn kernels

- Fresh cilantro for garnish

**Instructions:**

1. In a bowl, toss shrimp with Cajun seasoning.

2. Heat olive oil in a skillet over medium-high heat.

3. Cook shrimp for 2-3 minutes per side or until opaque.

4. In a bowl, assemble brown rice, diced bell pepper, diced red onion, and corn.

5. Top with Cajun shrimp.

6. Garnish with fresh cilantro before serving.

**Nutritional Information:**

- Calories: 320

- Protein: 25g

- Fat: 15g

- Carbohydrates: 30g

- Fiber: 5g

# Chapter 8: Dessert

## Chocolate Avocado Mousse

**Prep Time:** 15 minutes
**Cook Time:** 0 minutes
**Serving Size:** 4

**Ingredients:**

- 2 ripe avocados

- 1/4 cup unsweetened cocoa powder

- 1/4 cup honey

- 1 teaspoon vanilla extract

- Pinch of salt

- Fresh berries for garnish

**Instructions:**

1. In a blender, combine avocados, cocoa powder, honey, vanilla extract, and a pinch of salt.

2. Blend until smooth and creamy.

3. Refrigerate for at least 1 hour before serving.

4. Garnish with fresh berries before serving.

**Nutritional Information:**

- Calories: 180

- Protein: 3g

- Fat: 12g

- Carbohydrates: 20g

- Fiber: 6g

**Prep Time:** 5 minutes (plus overnight chilling)

**Cook Time:** 0 minutes

**Serving Size:** 4

**Ingredients:**

- 1/2 cup chia seeds

- 2 cups coconut milk

- 2 tablespoons maple syrup

- 1 teaspoon vanilla extract

- Shredded coconut for garnish

**Instructions:**

1. In a bowl, mix chia seeds, coconut milk, maple syrup, and vanilla extract.

2. Cover and refrigerate overnight or for at least 4 hours.

3. Stir well before serving.

4. Garnish with shredded coconut.

**Nutritional Information:**

- Calories: 160

- Protein: 4g

- Fat: 10g

- Carbohydrates: 15g

- Fiber: 8g

**Prep Time:** 10 minutes
**Cook Time:** 30 minutes
**Serving Size:** 4

**Ingredients:**

- 4 apples, cored and halved

- 1/4 cup chopped walnuts

- 2 tablespoons honey

- 1 teaspoon ground cinnamon

- Greek yogurt for serving

**Instructions:**

1. Preheat the oven to 350°F (180°C).

2. In a bowl, mix chopped walnuts, honey, and ground cinnamon.

3. Place apple halves on a baking sheet and fill each with the walnut mixture.

4. Bake for 30 minutes or until apples are tender.

5. Serve with a dollop of Greek yogurt.

**Nutritional Information:**

- Calories: 200

- Protein: 3g

- Fat: 8g

- Carbohydrates: 35g

- Fiber: 6g

**Prep Time:** 15 minutes

**Cook Time:** 0 minutes

**Serving Size:** 4

**Ingredients:**

- 2 cups mixed berries (strawberries, blueberries, raspberries)

- 1 cup almond yogurt

- 1/2 cup granola

- 1/4 cup sliced almonds

- Fresh mint for garnish

**Instructions:**

1. In serving glasses, layer mixed berries, almond yogurt, and granola.

2. Repeat the layers.

3. Top with sliced almonds and garnish with fresh mint.

4. Serve immediately.

**Nutritional Information:**

- Calories: 220

- Protein: 5g

- Fat: 10g

- Carbohydrates: 30g

- Fiber: 6g

Berry and Almond Parfait

# Mango Coconut Sorbet

**Prep Time:** 10 minutes (plus freezing time)
**Cook Time:** 0 minutes
**Serving Size:** 4

**Ingredients:**

- 2 cups frozen mango chunks

- 1/2 cup coconut milk

- 2 tablespoons lime juice

- Mint leaves for garnish

**Instructions:**

1. In a blender, combine frozen mango chunks, coconut milk, and lime juice.

2. Blend until smooth.

3. Transfer the mixture to a shallow dish and freeze for at least 4 hours.

4. Scoop and garnish with mint leaves before serving.

**Nutritional Information:**

- Calories: 160

- Protein: 2g

- Fat: 8g

- Carbohydrates: 25g

- Fiber: 3g

**Prep Time:** 15 minutes

**Cook Time:** 0 minutes

**Serving Size:** 10 bites

**Ingredients:**

- 1 cup rolled oats

- 1/2 cup pumpkin puree

- 1/4 cup almond butter

- 1/4 cup honey

- 1 teaspoon pumpkin spice

- 1/2 cup protein powder

- Chopped pecans for rolling

**Instructions:**

1. In a bowl, mix rolled oats, pumpkin puree, almond butter, honey, pumpkin spice, and protein powder.

2. Roll the mixture into bite-sized balls.

3. Roll each ball in chopped pecans to coat.

4. Refrigerate for at least 1 hour before serving.

**Nutritional Information:**

- Calories: 120

- Protein: 5g

- Fat: 6g

- Carbohydrates: 15g

- Fiber: 2g

# Lemon Blueberry Chia Muffins

**Prep Time:** 15 minutes
**Cook Time:** 20 minutes
**Serving Size:** 12 muffins

**Ingredients:**

- 2 cups almond flour

- 1/4 cup chia seeds

- 1 teaspoon baking powder

- 1/2 teaspoon baking soda

- Pinch of salt

- 1/4 cup coconut oil, melted

- 1/4 cup honey

- 3 eggs

- 1/4 cup almond milk

- Zest and juice of 1 lemon

- 1 cup blueberries

**Instructions:**

1. Preheat the oven to 350°F (180°C) and line a muffin tin with liners.

2. In a bowl, whisk together almond flour, chia seeds, baking powder, baking soda, and salt.

3. In another bowl, whisk together melted coconut oil, honey, eggs, almond milk, lemon zest, and lemon juice.

4. Combine wet and dry ingredients and fold in blueberries.

5. Spoon the batter into the muffin tin and bake for 20 minutes or until a toothpick comes out clean.

**Nutritional Information:**

- Calories: 180

- Protein: 6g

- Fat: 14g

- Carbohydrates: 12g

- Fiber: 3g

## Almond Butter Chocolate Chip Cookies

**Prep Time:** 10 minutes
**Cook Time:** 12 minutes
**Serving Size:** 16 cookies

**Ingredients:**

- 1 cup almond butter

- 1/2 cup coconut sugar

- 1 egg

- 1 teaspoon vanilla extract

- 1/2 teaspoon baking soda

- Pinch of salt

- 1/2 cup dark chocolate chips

**Instructions:**

1. Preheat the oven to 350°F (180°C) and line a baking sheet with parchment paper.

2. In a bowl, mix almond butter, coconut sugar, egg, vanilla extract, baking soda, and a pinch of salt.

3. Fold in dark chocolate chips.

4. Drop tablespoon-sized portions onto the prepared baking sheet.

5. Bake for 10-12 minutes or until the edges are golden.

**Nutritional Information:**

- Calories: 140

- Protein: 4g

- Fat: 10g

- Carbohydrates: 10g

- Fiber: 2g

**Prep Time:** 15 minutes
**Cook Time:** 25 minutes
**Serving Size:** 9 bars

**Ingredients:**

- 1 cup almond flour

- 1/4 cup coconut flour

- 1/4 cup coconut sugar

- 1/2 teaspoon baking powder

- Pinch of salt

- 1/4 cup coconut oil, melted

- 1 egg

- 1 teaspoon almond extract

- 1/2 cup raspberry jam

**Instructions:**

1. Preheat the oven to 350°F (180°C) and line a baking dish with parchment paper.

2. In a bowl, whisk together almond flour, coconut flour, coconut sugar, baking powder, and salt.

3. In another bowl, mix melted coconut oil, egg, and almond extract.

4. Combine wet and dry ingredients.

5. Spread half of the batter in the baking dish, top with raspberry jam, and cover with the remaining batter.

6. Bake for 25 minutes or until a toothpick comes out clean.

**Nutritional Information:**

- Calories: 180

- Protein: 4g

- Fat: 12g

- Carbohydrates: 15g

- Fiber: 3g

## Cinnamon Pecan Baked Pears

**Prep Time:** 10 minutes
**Cook Time:** 30 minutes
**Serving Size:** 4

**Ingredients:**

- 4 ripe but firm pears, halved and cored

- 1/4 cup chopped pecans

- 2 tablespoons honey

- 1 teaspoon ground cinnamon

- Greek yogurt for serving

**Instructions:**

1. Preheat the oven to 375°F (190°C).

2. Place pear halves in a baking dish.

3. In a bowl, mix chopped pecans, honey, and ground cinnamon.

4. Fill each pear half with the pecan mixture.

5. Bake for 30 minutes or until pears are tender.

6. Serve with a dollop of Greek yogurt.

**Nutritional Information:**

- Calories: 180

- Protein: 2g

- Fat: 8g

- Carbohydrates: 30g

- Fiber: 6g

**Prep Time:** 10 minutes (plus chilling time)

**Cook Time:** 0 minutes

**Serving Size:** 4

**Ingredients:**

- 1/2 cup chia seeds

- 2 cups unsweetened almond milk

- 2 tablespoons honey

- 1 teaspoon vanilla extract

- Mixed berries for topping

**Instructions:**

1. In a bowl, combine chia seeds, almond milk, honey, and vanilla extract.

2. Whisk well and refrigerate for at least 4 hours or overnight.

3. Stir before serving and top with mixed berries.

**Nutritional Information:**

- Calories: 150

- Protein: 4g

- Fat: 8g

- Carbohydrates: 18g

- Fiber: 8g

**Prep Time:** 5 minutes
**Cook Time:** 15 minutes
**Serving Size:** 6

**Ingredients:**

- 2 cups raw almonds

- 2 tablespoons unsweetened cocoa powder

- 1 tablespoon coconut sugar

- 1/2 teaspoon vanilla extract

- Pinch of sea salt

**Instructions:**

1. Preheat the oven to 325°F (160°C) and line a baking sheet with parchment paper.

2. In a bowl, mix almonds, cocoa powder, coconut sugar, vanilla extract, and a pinch of sea salt.

3. Spread the almonds on the baking sheet and bake for 15 minutes, stirring halfway through.

4. Let cool before serving.

**Nutritional Information:**

- Calories: 200

- Protein: 7g

- Fat: 17g

- Carbohydrates: 7g

- Fiber: 5g

**Prep Time:** 15 minutes

**Cook Time:** 12 minutes

**Serving Size:** 12 cookies

**Ingredients:**

- 2 ripe bananas, mashed

- 1 cup old-fashioned oats

- 1/4 cup chopped walnuts

- 1/4 cup raisins

- 1 teaspoon cinnamon

- 1/2 teaspoon vanilla extract

**Instructions:**

1. Preheat the oven to 350°F (180°C) and line a baking sheet with parchment paper.

2. In a bowl, mix mashed bananas, oats, chopped walnuts, raisins, cinnamon, and vanilla extract.

3. Drop spoonfuls of the mixture onto the baking sheet.

4. Bake for 12 minutes or until golden brown.

**Nutritional Information:**

- Calories: 90

- Protein: 2g

- Fat: 3g

- Carbohydrates: 15g

- Fiber: 2g

**Prep Time:** 15 minutes

**Cook Time:** 0 minutes

**Serving Size:** 4

**Ingredients:**

- 1 cup dark chocolate chips

- 2 cups fresh strawberries, washed and dried

**Instructions:**

1. Melt dark chocolate chips in a microwave-safe bowl in 30-second intervals, stirring until smooth.

2. Dip each strawberry into the melted chocolate, coating them halfway.

3. Place on a parchment-lined tray and let cool until the chocolate hardens.

**Nutritional Information:**

- Calories: 150

- Protein: 2g

- Fat: 8g

- Carbohydrates: 20g

- Fiber: 4g

**Prep Time:** 10 minutes
**Cook Time:** 0 minutes
**Serving Size:** 4

**Ingredients:**

- 2 cups Greek yogurt

- 2 peaches, sliced

- 1/2 cup almond slices

- 2 tablespoons honey

- Granola for topping

**Instructions:**

1. In serving glasses, layer Greek yogurt, sliced peaches, almond slices, and drizzle with honey.

2. Repeat the layers.

3. Top with granola before serving.

**Nutritional Information:**

- Calories: 220

- Protein: 15g

- Fat: 10g

- Carbohydrates: 20g

- Fiber: 3g

Peach and Almond Yogurt Parfait

# Chapter 9: Soup and stews



## Turmeric Lentil Soup

**Prep Time:** 15 minutes
**Cook Time:** 40 minutes
**Serving Size:** 6

**Ingredients:**

- 1 cup dry lentils, rinsed

- 1 onion, chopped

- 2 carrots, diced

- 2 celery stalks, chopped

- 3 cloves garlic, minced

- 1 tablespoon olive oil

- 1 teaspoon ground turmeric

- 1 teaspoon ground cumin

- 1/2 teaspoon smoked paprika

- 6 cups vegetable broth

- Salt and pepper to taste

- Fresh cilantro for garnish

**Instructions:**

1. In a large pot, sauté onions, carrots, celery, and garlic in olive oil until softened.

2. Add turmeric, cumin, smoked paprika, lentils, and vegetable broth.

3. Bring to a boil, then reduce heat and simmer for 30-40 minutes or until lentils are tender.

4. Season with salt and pepper.

5. Garnish with fresh cilantro before serving.

**Nutritional Information:**

- Calories: 220

- Protein: 13g

- Fat: 3g

- Carbohydrates: 35g

- Fiber: 12g

## Roasted Butternut Squash Soup

**Prep Time:** 20 minutes
**Cook Time:** 40 minutes
**Serving Size:** 6

**Ingredients:**

- 1 medium butternut squash, peeled and cubed

- 1 onion, diced

- 2 carrots, chopped

- 2 apples, cored and sliced

- 3 cups vegetable broth

- 1 teaspoon ground cinnamon

- 1/2 teaspoon ground nutmeg

- Salt and pepper to taste

- Greek yogurt for garnish

- Chopped chives for garnish

**Instructions:**

1. Preheat the oven to 400°F (200°C).

2. Roast butternut squash, onion, carrots, and apples on a baking sheet until tender (about 30 minutes).

3. Transfer roasted vegetables and apples to a pot, add vegetable broth, cinnamon, nutmeg, salt, and pepper.

4. Simmer for 10 minutes.

5. Blend until smooth.

6. Serve with a dollop of Greek yogurt and chopped chives.

**Nutritional Information:**

- Calories: 180
- Protein: 5g
- Fat: 1g
- Carbohydrates: 45g
- Fiber: 8g

**Prep Time:** 15 minutes

**Cook Time:** 35 minutes

**Serving Size:** 6

**Ingredients:**

- 1 cup quinoa, rinsed

- 1 onion, chopped

- 3 cloves garlic, minced

- 2 carrots, sliced

- 2 zucchinis, diced

- 1 bell pepper, chopped

- 1 can (15 oz) diced tomatoes

- 4 cups vegetable broth

- 1 teaspoon dried oregano

- 1 teaspoon ground cumin

- Salt and pepper to taste

- Fresh parsley for garnish

**Instructions:**

1. In a large pot, sauté onion and garlic until softened.

2. Add quinoa, carrots, zucchinis, bell pepper, diced tomatoes, vegetable broth, oregano, cumin, salt, and pepper.

3. Bring to a boil, then simmer for 25-30 minutes or until quinoa is cooked.

4. Adjust seasoning if needed.

5. Garnish with fresh parsley before serving.

**Nutritional Information:**

- Calories: 240

- Protein: 9g

- Fat: 3g

- Carbohydrates: 45g

- Fiber: 7g

## Spicy Black Bean Soup

**Prep Time:** 15 minutes
**Cook Time:** 30 minutes
**Serving Size:** 6

**Ingredients:**

- 2 cans (15 oz each) black beans, drained and rinsed

- 1 onion, diced

- 2 bell peppers, diced

- 3 cloves garlic, minced

- 1 jalapeño, seeded and chopped

- 1 tablespoon olive oil

- 1 teaspoon ground cumin

- 1 teaspoon chili powder

- 4 cups vegetable broth

- 1 cup corn kernels (fresh or frozen)

- Salt and pepper to taste

- Avocado slices for garnish

- Fresh cilantro for garnish

**Instructions:**

1. In a large pot, sauté onion, bell peppers, garlic, and jalapeño in olive oil until softened.

2. Add black beans, cumin, chili powder, vegetable broth, and corn.

3. Bring to a boil, then simmer for 20-25 minutes.

4. Season with salt and pepper.

5. Serve with avocado slices and fresh cilantro.

**Nutritional Information:**

- Calories: 230

- Protein: 10g

- Fat: 5g

- Carbohydrates: 40g

- Fiber: 12g

**Prep Time:** 20 minutes
**Cook Time:** 45 minutes
**Serving Size:** 6

**Ingredients:**

- 1 cup pearl barley, rinsed

- 1 onion, finely chopped

- 3 carrots, diced

- 3 celery stalks, sliced

- 8 oz mushrooms, sliced

- 3 cloves garlic, minced

- 1 tablespoon olive oil

- 8 cups vegetable broth

- 1 teaspoon dried thyme

- Salt and pepper to taste

- Fresh parsley for garnish

**Instructions:**

1. In a large pot, sauté onion, carrots, celery, mushrooms, and garlic in olive oil until vegetables are tender.

2. Add pearl barley, vegetable broth, thyme, salt, and pepper.

3. Bring to a boil, then reduce heat and simmer for 35-40 minutes or until barley is cooked.

4. Adjust seasoning if needed.

5. Garnish with fresh parsley before serving.

**Nutritional Information:**

- Calories: 260

- Protein: 8g

- Fat: 4g

- Carbohydrates: 50g

- Fiber: 10g

## Cauliflower and Leek Chowder

**Prep Time:** 15 minutes
**Cook Time:** 35 minutes
**Serving Size:** 6

**Ingredients:**

- 1 cauliflower, chopped

- 2 leeks, sliced

- 3 potatoes, peeled and diced

- 2 cloves garlic, minced

- 2 tablespoons olive oil

- 4 cups vegetable broth

- 1 teaspoon dried thyme

- 1 cup unsweetened almond milk

- Salt and pepper to taste

- Chopped green onions for garnish

**Instructions:**

1. In a large pot, sauté cauliflower, leeks, potatoes, and garlic in olive oil until vegetables are slightly browned.

2. Add vegetable broth, thyme, salt, and pepper.

3. Simmer for 25-30 minutes or until vegetables are tender.

4. Blend the soup until smooth.

5. Stir in almond milk.

6. Garnish with chopped green onions before serving.

**Nutritional Information:**

- Calories: 220

- Protein: 6g

- Fat: 6g

- Carbohydrates: 40g

- Fiber: 8g

## Red Lentil and Spinach Stew

**Prep Time:** 15 minutes
**Cook Time:** 25 minutes
**Serving Size:** 6

**Ingredients:**

- 1 cup red lentils, rinsed

- 1 onion, chopped

- 3 carrots, sliced

- 4 cups vegetable broth

- 1 can (14 oz) diced tomatoes

- 2 cups fresh spinach

- 2 teaspoons ground cumin

- 1 teaspoon smoked paprika

- Salt and pepper to taste

- Lemon wedges for serving

**Instructions:**

1. In a pot, combine red lentils, onion, carrots, vegetable broth, diced tomatoes, cumin, smoked paprika, salt, and pepper.

2. Bring to a boil, then simmer for 20-25 minutes or until lentils are cooked.

3. Stir in fresh spinach until wilted.

4. Adjust seasoning if needed.

5. Serve with lemon wedges.

**Nutritional Information:**

- Calories: 200

- Protein: 10g

- Fat: 2g

- Carbohydrates: 35g

- Fiber: 12g

## Sweet Potato and Kale Soup

**Prep Time:** 20 minutes
**Cook Time:** 30 minutes
**Serving Size:** 6

**Ingredients:**

- 2 large sweet potatoes, peeled and diced

- 1 onion, diced

- 3 cloves garlic, minced

- 1 bunch kale, stems removed and leaves chopped

- 1 can (15 oz) white beans, drained and rinsed

- 4 cups vegetable broth

- 1 teaspoon ground coriander

- 1/2 teaspoon smoked paprika

- Salt and pepper to taste

- Greek yogurt for garnish

**Instructions:**

1. In a large pot, sauté sweet potatoes, onion, and garlic until onions are translucent.

2. Add kale, white beans, vegetable broth, ground coriander, smoked paprika, salt, and pepper.

3. Simmer for 20-25 minutes or until sweet potatoes are tender.

4. Adjust seasoning if needed.

5. Serve with a dollop of Greek yogurt.

**Nutritional Information:**

- Calories: 230

- Protein: 8g

- Fat: 1g

- Carbohydrates: 50g

- Fiber: 10g

## Tomato Basil Quinoa Soup

**Prep Time:** 15 minutes
**Cook Time:** 25 minutes
**Serving Size:** 6

**Ingredients:**

- 1 cup quinoa, rinsed

- 1 onion, chopped

- 3 carrots, sliced

- 3 cloves garlic, minced

- 1 can (28 oz) crushed tomatoes

- 4 cups vegetable broth

- 1 teaspoon dried basil

- 1/2 teaspoon dried oregano

- Salt and pepper to taste

- Fresh basil leaves for garnish

**Instructions:**

1. In a pot, sauté onion, carrots, and garlic until softened.

2. Add quinoa, crushed tomatoes, vegetable broth, dried basil, dried oregano, salt, and pepper.

3. Bring to a boil, then simmer for 20-25 minutes or until quinoa is cooked.

4. Adjust seasoning if needed.

5.  Garnish with fresh basil leaves before serving.

    **Nutritional Information:**

- Calories: 250

- Protein: 10g

- Fat: 3g

- Carbohydrates: 45g

- Fiber: 8g

**Prep Time:** 20 minutes
**Cook Time:** 40 minutes
**Serving Size:** 6

**Ingredients:**

- 2 cans (15 oz each) chickpeas, drained and rinsed

- 1 onion, diced

- 3 cloves garlic, minced

- 1 bell pepper, chopped

- 1 zucchini, diced

- 1 can (14 oz) coconut milk

- 2 tablespoons red curry paste

- 4 cups vegetable broth

- 1 tablespoon soy sauce

- 1 tablespoon maple syrup

- Fresh cilantro for garnish

**Instructions:**

1. In a pot, sauté onion, garlic, bell pepper, and zucchini until vegetables are tender.

2. Add chickpeas, coconut milk, red curry paste, vegetable broth, soy sauce, and maple syrup.

3. Simmer for 30-35 minutes.

4. Adjust seasoning if needed.

5. Garnish with fresh cilantro before serving.

**Nutritional Information:**

- Calories: 280

- Protein: 12g

- Fat: 10g

- Carbohydrates: 40g

- Fiber: 10g

## Lemon Garlic Chickpea Stew

**Prep Time:** 15 minutes
**Cook Time:** 30 minutes
**Serving Size:** 6

**Ingredients:**

- 2 cans (15 oz each) chickpeas, drained and rinsed

- 1 onion, chopped

- 4 cloves garlic, minced

- 1 lemon, juiced and zested

- 1 can (14 oz) diced tomatoes

- 4 cups vegetable broth

- 1 teaspoon dried thyme

- 1/2 teaspoon ground coriander

- Salt and pepper to taste

- Fresh parsley for garnish

**Instructions:**

1. In a pot, sauté onion and garlic until softened.

2. Add chickpeas, lemon juice and zest, diced tomatoes, vegetable broth, thyme, ground coriander, salt, and pepper.

3. Simmer for 25-30 minutes.

4. Adjust seasoning if needed.

5. Garnish with fresh parsley before serving.

**Nutritional Information:**

- Calories: 220

- Protein: 10g

- Fat: 3g

- Carbohydrates: 40g

- Fiber: 10g

## Cabbage and White Bean Soup

**Prep Time:** 20 minutes
**Cook Time:** 35 minutes
**Serving Size:** 6

**Ingredients:**

- 1 small head cabbage, shredded

- 1 onion, diced

- 3 carrots, sliced

- 3 celery stalks, chopped

- 2 cans (15 oz each) cannellini beans, drained and rinsed

- 4 cups vegetable broth

- 1 teaspoon Italian seasoning

- 1/2 teaspoon red pepper flakes

- Salt and pepper to taste

- Grated Parmesan cheese for garnish

**Instructions:**

1. In a large pot, sauté onion, carrots, and celery until softened.

2. Add shredded cabbage, cannellini beans, vegetable broth, Italian seasoning, red pepper flakes, salt, and pepper.

3. Simmer for 30-35 minutes.

4. Adjust seasoning if needed.

5. Serve with a sprinkle of grated Parmesan cheese.

**Nutritional Information:**

- Calories: 180

- Protein: 8g

- Fat: 2g

- Carbohydrates: 35g

- Fiber: 12g

## Miso Vegetable Soup

**Prep Time:** 15 minutes
**Cook Time:** 20 minutes
**Serving Size:** 4

**Ingredients:**

- 4 cups vegetable broth

- 2 tablespoons miso paste

- 1 carrot, julienned

- 1 zucchini, spiralized

- 1 cup shiitake mushrooms, sliced

- 2 green onions, sliced

- 1 tablespoon soy sauce

- 1 teaspoon sesame oil

- Seaweed sheets for garnish

**Instructions:**

1. In a pot, whisk together vegetable broth and miso paste until well combined.

2. Bring to a gentle simmer.

3. Add carrot, zucchini, shiitake mushrooms, green onions, soy sauce, and sesame oil.

4. Simmer for 15-20 minutes.

5. Adjust seasoning if needed.

6. Garnish with seaweed sheets before serving.

**Nutritional Information:**

- Calories: 120

- Protein: 6g

- Fat: 4g

- Carbohydrates: 18g

- Fiber: 5g

## Cajun Black-Eyed Pea Soup

**Prep Time:** 15 minutes
**Cook Time:** 40 minutes
**Serving Size:** 6

**Ingredients:**

- 2 cans (15 oz each) black-eyed peas, drained and rinsed

- 1 onion, chopped

- 2 bell peppers, diced

- 3 celery stalks, sliced

- 3 cloves garlic, minced

- 1 tablespoon olive oil

- 1 tablespoon Cajun seasoning

- 1 can (14 oz) diced tomatoes

- 4 cups vegetable broth

- Salt and pepper to taste

- Fresh thyme for garnish

**Instructions:**

1. In a pot, sauté onion, bell peppers, celery, and garlic in olive oil until softened.

2. Add Cajun seasoning, black-eyed peas, diced tomatoes, and vegetable broth.

3. Bring to a boil, then simmer for 30-35 minutes.

4. Season with salt and pepper.

5.  Garnish with fresh thyme before serving.

    **Nutritional Information:**

- Calories: 250

- Protein: 12g

- Fat: 4g

- Carbohydrates: 40g

- Fiber: 12g

# Thai Coconut Pumpkin Soup

**Prep Time:** 20 minutes
**Cook Time:** 30 minutes
**Serving Size:** 4

**Ingredients:**

- 2 cups pumpkin puree

- 1 can (14 oz) coconut milk

- 1 onion, chopped

- 2 carrots, sliced

- 2 tablespoons red curry paste

- 1 tablespoon fresh ginger, minced

- 4 cups vegetable broth

- 1 tablespoon soy sauce

- 1 tablespoon lime juice

- Fresh cilantro for garnish

**Instructions:**

1. In a pot, combine pumpkin puree, coconut milk, onion, carrots, red curry paste, ginger, vegetable broth, soy sauce, and lime juice.

2. Bring to a simmer and cook for 25-30 minutes.

3. Adjust seasoning if needed.

4. Garnish with fresh cilantro before serving.

**Nutritional Information:**

- Calories: 230

- Protein: 5g

- Fat: 15g

- Carbohydrates: 25g

- Fiber: 8g

# Conclusion

Congratulations on starting your journey with "The Galveston Diet Cookbook for Beginners"! As you explore the delightful recipes in this cookbook, you will have not only made steps toward a better living, but also accepted the concepts that distinguish The Galveston Diet.

The Galveston Diet is more than just fueling your body; it's a comprehensive strategy that recognizes the link between nutrition, hormone balance, and general health. By using recipes from this cookbook, you've given yourself the ability to make informed nutritional decisions that prioritize nutrient-dense and healthful products.

Whether you're enjoying the vibrant flavors of the breakfast options, indulging in nutritious snacks and appetizers, relishing the goodness of vegetables and sides, savoring the richness of fish and seafood, delighting in the heartiness of beef, pork, and lamb dishes, or treating yourself to the sweet endings of desserts, each recipe adheres to The Galveston Diet's principles.

Remember that this journey is about more than simply the food you eat; it's about nourishing your body, balancing hormones, and promoting overall health. As you experiment with these recipes, remember to listen to your body, pay attention to portion proportions, and appreciate the nutritious power of each meal.

I wish you a fulfilling and delightful trip with The Galveston Diet Cookbook. May your meals be pleasant, your health thrive, and your well-being prosper!

As you continue your culinary journey with "The Galveston Diet Cookbook for Beginners," keep in mind that it is more than just a collection of dishes; it is also a guide to a balanced and healthy lifestyle. The principles provided in the cookbook are intended to help you attain long-term health advantages.

Explore the nutrient-dense recipes available, experiment with flavors, and experience the delight of making meals that not only satisfy your taste buds but also benefit your overall health. This cookbook's dishes are designed to correspond with The Galveston Diet concept, which emphasizes whole, unadulterated foods and mindful eating.

Along with the tasty meals, consider adding other aspects of The Galveston Diet into your daily routine, such as staying active, minimizing stress, and prioritizing quality sleep. These behavioral aspects supplement the nutritional part of the diet, leading to a more comprehensive approach to well-being.

As you embark on this road, keep in mind that it is absolutely okay to indulge on occasion. The Galveston Diet aims to foster a long-term and healthy relationship with food, allowing for flexibility while prioritizing nourishment.

May your experience with "The Galveston Diet Cookbook for Beginners" be filled with culinary joys, better health, and a renewed awareness for the good impact that conscious eating can have on your life. Cheers to your health and happiness!